Pathological Gambling

A Clinical Guide to Treatment

D0250870

Pathological Gambling

A Clinical Guide to Treatment

Edited by

Jon E. Grant, J.D., M.D., M.P.H.
Marc N. Potenza, M.D., Ph.D.

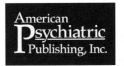

Washington, DC
London, England

Note: The authors have worked to ensure that all information in this book is accurate at the time of publication and consistent with general psychiatric and medical standards, and that information concerning drug dosages, schedules, and routes of administration is accurate at the time of publication and consistent with standards set by the U.S. Food and Drug Administration and the general medical community. As medical research and practice continue to advance, however, therapeutic standards may change. Moreover, specific situations may require a specific therapeutic response not included in this book. For these reasons and because human and mechanical errors sometimes occur, we recommend that readers follow the advice of physicians directly involved in their care or the care of a member of their family.

Copyright © 2004 American Psychiatric Publishing, Inc.
ALL RIGHTS RESERVED

Manufactured in the United States of America on acid-free paper
08 07 06 05 04   5 4 3 2 1
First Edition

Typeset in Adobe's Berling Roman and Frutiger55 Roman

American Psychiatric Publishing, Inc.
1000 Wilson Boulevard
Arlington, VA 22209-3901
www.appi.org

Library of Congress Cataloging-in-Publication Data
Pathological gambling : a clinical guide to treatment / edited by Jon E. Grant,
    Marc N. Potenza.—1st ed.
        p. ; cm.
    Includes bibliographical references and index.
    ISBN 1-58562-129-3 (pbk. : alk. paper)
    1. Compulsive gambling. 2. Compulsive gambling—Treatment.
3. Compulsive gamblers—Rehabilitation. I. Grant, Jon E. II. Potenza, Marc N.,
    1965–
    [DNLM: 1. Gambling—psychology. 2. Impulsive Control Disorders—
therapy. WM 190 P2968 2004]
RC569.5.G35P375 2004
616.85′84106—dc22

                                                                        2004050257

British Library Cataloguing in Publication Data
A CIP record is available from the British Library.

Contents

Part I
Public Health and Epidemiology

Part II
Clinical Characteristics

Part III
Etiology

Part IV
Prevention and Treatment

Contributors

Kenneth Abrams, Ph.D.
Assistant Professor of Psychology, Psychology Department, University of Richmond, Richmond, Virginia

Tami R. Argo, Pharm.D.
Postdoctoral Fellow, University of Iowa College of Pharmacy, Iowa City, Iowa

Donald W. Black, M.D.
Professor, Department of Psychiatry, University of Iowa, Roy J. and Lucille A. Carver College of Medicine, Iowa City, Iowa

Carlos Blanco, M.D., Ph.D.
Assistant Clinical Professor of Psychiatry, New York State Psychiatric Institute/Columbia University, New York, New York

Linda B. Cottler, Ph.D.
Professor of Epidemiology in Psychiatry, Washington University School of Medicine, St. Louis, Missouri

Renee M. Cunningham-Williams, Ph.D., M.P.E.
Research Assistant Professor of Social Work in Psychiatry, Department of Psychiatry, Washington University School of Medicine, St. Louis, Missouri

Jeffrey L. Derevensky, Ph.D.

Professor of School/Applied Child Psychology and Associate Professor, Department of Psychiatry, McGill University, Montreal, Quebec, Canada

Rani A. Desai, M.P.H., Ph.D.

Assistant Professor of Psychiatry, Epidemiology, and Public Health, Yale University School of Medicine, West Haven, Connecticut

Laurie Dickson, M.A.

Doctoral Student, School/Applied Child Psychology, McGill University, Montreal, Quebec, Canada

Seth A. Eisen, M.D.

Staff Physician, St. Louis VA Medical Center; Professor of Internal Medicine and Psychiatry, Washington University School of Medicine, St. Louis, Missouri

G. Ron Frisch, Ph.D., C.Psych.

Professor of Psychology, University of Windsor, Windsor, Ontario, Canada

Richard Govoni, Ph.D.

Research Director, Problem Gambling Research Group and Assistant Professor (Adjunct), Department of Psychology, University of Windsor, Windsor, Ontario, Canada

Jon E. Grant, J.D., M.D., M.P.H.

Assistant Professor of Psychiatry and Human Behavior, Brown Medical School and Director, Impulse Control Disorders Clinic, Butler Hospital, Providence, Rhode Island

Mark D. Griffiths, Ph.D., C.Psychol.

Professor of Gambling Studies, Psychology Division, Nottingham Trent University, Nottingham, England

Rina Gupta, Ph.D.

Assistant Professor of School/Applied Child Psychology, McGill University, Montreal, Quebec, Canada

David C. Hodgins, Ph.D.
Professor, Department of Psychology, University of Calgary, Calgary, Alberta, Canada

Eric Hollander, M.D.
Professor of Psychiatry and Director, Compulsive, Impulsive and Anxiety Disorders Program, Department of Psychiatry, Mount Sinai School of Medicine, New York, New York

Angela Ibáñez, M.D., Ph.D.
Department of Psychiatry, Hospital Ramón y Cajal, Universidad de Alcalá de Henares, Madrid, Spain

Alicia Kaplan, M.D.
Research Fellow, Compulsive, Impulsive and Anxiety Disorders Program, Department of Psychiatry, Mount Sinai School of Medicine, New York, New York

Rachel Kidman
Research Assistant, Division on Addictions, Harvard Medical School, Boston, Massachusetts

Suck Won Kim, M.D.
Associate Professor of Psychiatry, Department of Psychiatry, University of Minnesota, Minneapolis, Minnesota

Matt G. Kushner, Ph.D.
Associate Professor of Psychiatry, Department of Psychiatry, University of Minnesota, Minneapolis, Minnesota

Paula Moreyra, M.A.
Anxiety Disorders Clinic, New York State Psychiatric Institute

Stefano Pallanti, M.D.
Associate Professor of Psychiatry, University of Florence, Florence, Italy; Adjunct Associate Professor of Psychiatry, Mount Sinai School of Medicine, New York, New York

Nancy M. Petry, Ph.D.
Professor, Department of Psychiatry, University of Connecticut Health Center, Farmington, Connecticut

Marc N. Potenza, M.D., Ph.D.

Assistant Professor of Psychiatry, Yale University School of Medicine, New Haven, Connecticut

Jerónimo Saiz-Ruiz, M.D., Ph.D.

Department of Psychiatry, Hospital Ramón y Cajal, Universidad de Alcalá de Henares, Madrid, Spain

Howard J. Shaffer, Ph.D., C.A.S.

Associate Professor and Director, Division on Addictions, Harvard Medical School; Department of Psychiatry, The Cambridge Hospital, Boston, Massachusetts

Kamini R. Shah, M.H.S.

Study Coordinator, St. Louis VA Medical Center; Data Analyst, Washington University School of Medicine, St. Louis, Missouri

Randy Stinchfield, Ph.D., L.P.

Clinical Psychologist and Assistant Professor, Department of Psychiatry, University of Minnesota, Minneapolis, Minnesota

Ken C. Winters, Ph.D.

Associate Professor of Psychiatry, Department of Psychiatry, University of Minnesota, Minneapolis, Minnesota

Sharon B. Womack, Ph.D., M.P.E.

Postdoctoral Trainee, Department of Psychiatry, Washington University School of Medicine, St. Louis, Missouri

Introduction

Jon E. Grant, J.D., M.D., M.P.H.
Marc N. Potenza, M.D., Ph.D.

In the last 5 years, the volume of research on pathological gambling has grown significantly. Thus, as a textbook devoted exclusively to pathological gambling, this volume reflects an exciting moment in the history of pathological gambling research. Because of this research, clinicians now have available an array of treatment options that can appreciably improve the lives of patients with pathological gambling.

The study of pathological gambling is important from both clinical and research perspectives. Pathological gambling is a prevalent disorder (with prevalence estimates surpassing those for bipolar disorder and schizophrenia) that is associated with significant morbidity (decreased self-esteem, comorbid substance use disorders, financial and legal difficulties, stress on relationships and families, and suicidality). In recent years, the understanding of the phenomenology, epidemiology, neurobiology, psychology, and treatment of this disorder has rapidly increased. Unfortunately, although many clinicians encounter pathological gamblers (elevated rates of pathological gambling are observed in patients with mental health disorders), clinicians often do not diagnose pathological gambling and are frequently unaware of the treatment options for the disorder.

Many clinicians are also unaware of the personal and social consequences of pathological gambling. This lack of awareness in turn often leads physicians to ignore pathological gambling evaluations in both psychiatric and primary care settings. Pathological gambling has significant public health implications, and Shaffer and Kidman (Chapter 1, "Gambling and the Public Health") provide an initial review of definitions for recreational, problem, and pathological gambling; examine the relationship between the different levels of gambling severity; and explore the effects of gambling on societal, familial, and individual health and well-being. An understanding of the prevalence of pathological gambling (Chapter 2, "Epidemiology") will help clinicians to realize how likely they are to encounter the problem. Assessment instruments that are useful in diagnosing pathological gambling and monitoring symptom change are discussed (Chapter 14, "Screening and Assessment Instruments") and are provided for the clinician in the Appendixes.

The primary purpose of this book is to document the clinical phenomenology, etiology, and treatment of pathological gambling. Current clinical approaches that are most likely to lead to early identification, symptom remission, and maintenance of improvement are highlighted. Argo and Black (Chapter 3, "Clinical Characteristics") provide a comprehensive description of the symptoms and sequelae of pathological gambling. The book also provides contributions on how pathological gambling differs in the adolescent population (Chapter 5, "Adolescents and Young Adults"), among older adults (Chapter 6, "Older Adults"), and between men and women (Chapter 7, "Gender Differences").

Much of the treatment literature on pathological gambling has been based on different theories regarding the categorization of the disorder. Treatment has varied depending on whether pathological gambling has been characterized as an obsessive-compulsive spectrum disorder, an affective spectrum disorder, an addiction, or an impulse control disorder. As discussed by Moreyra and colleagues, a range of evidence indicates that pathological gambling often shares important features with all of these disorders (Chapter 4, "Categorization").

To further enhance treatment options, both clinicians and researchers look to possible psychological and behavioral etiologies, as well as to a deeper understanding of possible neurobiological underpinnings. Therefore, these two important realms of explanations for the behavior of pathological gambling are examined. Abrams and Kushner (Chapter 8, "Behavioral Understanding") discuss behavioral, cognitive, and dispositional theories of the etiology of pathological gambling and provide an association between psychological models and neurobiological systems that have been linked to pathological gambling. To augment the psychological basis for pathological gambling, Shah and colleagues (Chapter 9, "Biological Basis for Pathological Gambling") examine the evidence that supports the involvement of the noradrenergic, serotonergic, dopaminergic, and opioidergic systems, as well as familial and inherited factors in pathological gambling. The psychological and biological understanding of pathological gambling may be useful in understanding a range of addictive and impulsive disorders.

Although effective treatments for pathological gambling currently exist, with this book we seek to enhance clinicians' abilities to identify and provide early intervention for individuals with pathological gambling. Toward that end, Potenza and Griffiths (Chapter 10, "Prevention Efforts and the Role of the Clinician") provide information regarding the important role for the clinician in prevention efforts. These authors argue for close communication between mental health professionals and generalist physicians in early identification and treatment. Adolescents and young adults have been consistently found to exhibit high rates of problem and pathological gambling (two to four times higher than in general adult populations). To address this issue, Derevensky and colleagues provide a prevention strategy tailored specifically for this age group (Chapter 11, "Prevention and Treatment of Adolescent Problem and Pathological Gambling").

Tremendous advances in the treatment of pathological gambling have been made within the past few years. As a result, clinicians caring for patients with pathological gambling have many treatment options at their disposal. Hodgins and Petry (Chapter 12, "Cognitive and Behavioral Treatments") discuss the current understanding of the behavioral treatment approaches and their effectiveness in helping individuals with pathological gambling. They evaluate the rationale behind, empirical support for, and practical aspects of a variety of behavioral interventions, including participation in 12-step programs, financial counseling, motivational interviewing, motivational enhancement, brief interventions, and cognitive-behavioral treatment. Furthermore, these authors discuss self-help–based and professional-based interventions targeting family members. In a related chapter, Hollander and colleagues (Chapter 13, "Pharmacological Treatments") discuss the rationale of the various pharmacological approaches to pathological gambling and review the current status of drug treatments. They examine the evidence for the use of serotonin reuptake inhibitors, serotonin receptor ($5\text{-}HT_2$) antagonists, mood stabilizers, opioid antagonists, and dopaminergic agents in treating pathological gambling.

In summary, pathological gambling is an important clinical condition that often results in significant personal difficulties for patients. As the chapters of this volume eloquently attest, extraordinary progress has been made regarding the epidemiology, phenomenology, comorbidity, and possible etiology of this disorder. Prevention and treatment interventions—including cognitive, behavioral, and pharmacological treatments—have made it possible for patients with pathological gambling to often find relief from this disabling disorder.

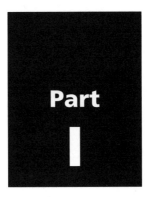

Part

I

Public Health and Epidemiology

Gambling and the Public Health

Howard J. Shaffer, Ph.D., C.A.S.
Rachel Kidman

Gambling studies is a young field poised at the edge of new terrain: the realm of public health. In this chapter, we anticipate this next stage of gambling-related research and encourage the use of an integrated public health approach to understanding gambling. A public health strategy will help scientists, makers of public policy, and communities deal with the costs and benefits of gambling. Specifically, in this chapter we summarize the epidemiological evidence about gambling, provide a description of the potential social impacts associated with gambling, and consider the implications for future research and policy.

Gambling: An Emerging Public Health Issue

For much of the history of gambling, observers considered intemperate betting to be a moral weakness (Quinn 1892). Gradually, people began to consider excessive gambling as a psychological or psychiatric problem (e.g., Freud 1928/1961; Jacobs 1989; Lindner 1950). Most recently, neurobiological views of intemperate gambling have started to emerge (Bergh et al. 1997; Blum et al. 2000; Breiter et al. 2001; Comings 1998; Hollander et al. 2000; Shaffer and Kidman 2003). Each of these perspectives emphasizes the individual gambler and his or her biopsychosocial attributes. Recently, researchers have been considering gambling from a public health standpoint (Korn and Shaffer 1999; Shaffer and Korn 2002; Shaffer et al. 2002; Skinner 1999). Approaching gambling from a public health perspective encourages the examination of health problems through a population-based lens. One benefit of this view is that it encourages consideration of health-related phenomena at a macro level of analysis that might not be available using more individual research approaches; consequently, there has been growing interest in viewing gambling from a public health perspective.

Gambling is a complex phenomenon; so too are its determinants. Just as the public health model of host, agent, and environment helped to advance the understanding of many communicable diseases, a similar public health strategy encourages us to examine the gambler's **individual-level characteristics, gambling activities,** and **social setting** (i.e., proximate and distal) within which the person gambles. The interaction among these factors is essential to the understanding of gambling and its effects.

Gambling activities involve risking something of value on the outcome of an event when the probability of winning or losing is determined by chance (Korn and Shaffer 1999). Forms of gambling are both formal and informal and range from individual to social activities. Like drugs, each form has unique attributes that can increase or decrease risk factors that are influential in the development of gambling-associated problems. Although providing descriptions of the different forms of gambling is beyond the scope of this chapter, readers should be aware that characteristics of different forms can influence the social setting and can contribute to the effects of gambling on individuals.

As a relatively new field, gambling research has been concerned primarily with describing the **individual-level characteristics** of gamblers. Since 1980, when the American Psychiatric Association first recognized intemperate gambling as a psychiatric disorder and named it *pathological gambling*, this approach to understanding gambling has emphasized psychobiological and cognitive factors. In addition, this strategy focused on the intrapersonal events associated with transitions from healthy to disordered gambling. Clinicians and researchers subscribing to this view developed a definition of disordered gambling and then created screening instruments based on the diagnostic criteria associated with these definitions.

Recently, gambling-related perspectives have shifted from a narrow focus on individual gamblers to a more expansive examination of the **social setting** (i.e., social factors that mediate gambling). Just as classification and description are the foundation for understanding a data set, epidemiological research represents the beginning phase for understanding population-based phenomena. Consequently, many gambling researchers have embarked on a course of epidemiological study to describe the distribution and determinants of gambling in the general population. In gambling studies, epidemiological evidence about the prevalence of gambling disorders has stabilized (e.g., Shaffer and Korn 2002), and a reliable description of the distribution of gambling involvement and gambling problems has emerged for many segments of the population. Thus, an integrative public health model encourages the era of general-population prevalence studies to end in favor of research based on population segments. This approach to the study of gambling encourages examination of the risk and protective factors that influence the transition from recreational to problem-related gambling and the identification of vulnerable demographic groups (e.g., ethnic differences associated with higher rates of gambling-related problems). Insights gained from study of a broad, population-based analysis will eventually necessitate a return to an individual level of analysis to ascertain how the social, economic, and cultural variables translate into health outcomes. Similarly, epidemiological studies of the general population will become relevant again when it becomes necessary to determine the success of new gambling-related policy, prevention, and treatment efforts.

To fully understand the impact of gambling on health, we must examine it from many different perspectives. The research path described above includes both an individualized medical approach and a population-based public health approach; each is essential to the study of gambling. These two approaches inform one another and encourage a recursive and integrated public health research strategy. Figure 1–1 illustrates an integrated view of public health research.

As shown in Figure 1–1, with each investigative cycle, observers gain a more precise definition and comprehensive understanding of gambling. Typically, the appropriate level of analysis expands to the population and narrows to the individual, depending on the current stage of research and its findings; sometimes, however, the study of gambling or other phenomena will move freely between these different levels of analysis.

Distribution of Gambling and Associated Problems

Growth of Gambling During the Modern Era

Three primary forces appear to be motivating the growth of gambling throughout North America: 1) the desire of governments to identify new

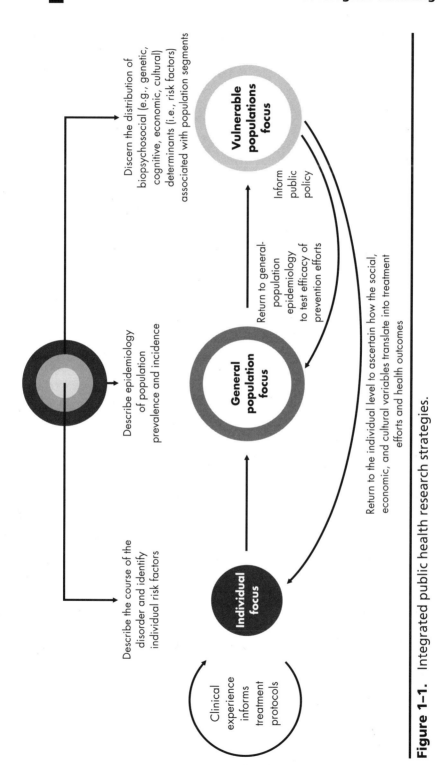

Figure 1–1.   Integrated public health research strategies.

sources of revenue without invoking new or higher taxes; 2) the development by tourism entrepreneurs of new destinations for entertainment and leisure; and 3) the rise of new technologies and forms of gambling (e.g., video lottery terminals, Powerball mega-lotteries, and Internet off-shore gambling) (Korn and Shaffer 1999).

In the United States between 1975 and 1999, participation trends show that adult gambling increased from 68% to 86%, gambling expenditures increased from 0.30% to 0.74% of personal income, and gambling patterns among women grew to resemble those of men (Gerstein et al. 1999).The most dramatic increase in lifetime gambling occurred in the 65 and above age group, in which it increased from 35% of older adults to 80% (Gerstein et al. 1999). Corporate profits in the gaming entertainment and related hospitality industries have soared. For example, 1996 figures for the leisure economy in the United States show that gross gambling revenues were $47.6 billion, which was greater than the $40.8 billion in combined revenues from film box office, recorded music, cruise ships, spectator sports, and live entertainment (Christiansen 1998). Gambling expenditures have continued to climb; in 2001, Americans made 303 million trips to casinos, resulting in casino-based revenue of $27.2 billion and contributing to gross gambling revenue of $63.3 billion. This represents an increase in revenue of one-third in just 5 years. Gambling revenue during 2001 was roughly equal to the amount spent on basic cable television, sound recordings, and movie box-office sales combined ($63.7 billion) (American Gaming Association 2002).

Spectrum of Individual Gambling Problems

During various periods in history, observers have recognized and characterized gambling-related problems in personal, social, and economic terms (e.g., greed, crime, and social costs). Public policy makers, scientists, and social critics have raised concerns that the rapid expansion of gambling during the latter part of the twentieth century has stimulated a variety of personal problems. The most apparent and perhaps best studied of these difficulties is disordered gambling. Gambling resides on a behavioral continuum that can range from none to excessive. Clinicians and researchers have transformed this quantitative continuum into discrete categories using many different and often confusing labels (e.g., at-risk, problem, subclinical, pathological, probable pathological, extremely pathological, in-transition, compulsive). Despite this confusing nomenclature, it is most common to consider disordered gambling dichotomously: clinical (i.e., excessive gambling that satisfies diagnostic criteria) and subclinical (i.e., gambling that is symptomatic but does not meet diagnostic criteria). Currently, pathological gambling represents a pattern of intemperate gambling that satisfies formal diagnostic criteria; there is no official term for subclinical gambling, although it is commonly referred to as problem gambling.

To respond to the complex definition and competing terms, gambling researchers and public policy makers have started adopting a system of levels: a type of public health tool commonly used to stratify the continuum of sickness to advance population-based understanding and research. For example, clinicians and researchers categorize burns, diabetes, and cancer using a level system (i.e., first-, second-, and third-degree burns; type 1 and type 2 diabetes; and so on). Gambling researchers use levels ranging from 0 to 4 to describe the prevalence of gambling-related behavior (Shaffer et al. 1997). Level 0 represents people who do not gamble. Level 1 represents people who gamble recreationally with no adverse consequences. When gambling behavior is associated with any of a wide range of negative consequences, however, it is classified as level 2 gambling, also referred to as problem gambling. Level 3 represents people with adverse consequences that are sufficiently serious and co-occurring as to meet the diagnostic criteria for pathological gambling. Finally, gamblers enter level 4 when they seek help for their problem regardless of the extent of their distress. One advantage of the level system is that it allows clinicians and researchers to avoid using pejorative language.

Estimates of pathological gambling among adults in the general population increased during the period between 1975 and 1999. The average prevalence estimate of current-year adult level 3 gamblers in the United States and Canada is 1.46%, and the corresponding prevalence estimate of level 2 gamblers is 2.54% (Shaffer and Hall 2001). When adjusted for extreme values, these estimates become 1.1% for level 3 and 2.2% for level 2 gamblers. The prevalence of disordered gambling is similar to the rate of other mental disorders and warrants comparable attention and resources.

Evidence suggests that gambling prevalence estimates for adults in the general population are relatively consistent across researchers, research strategies, and geographic space and time. Researchers from other countries have observed similar rates. For example, a study in Sweden estimated level 2 gambling to be 1.4% and level 3 gambling to be 0.6% (Volberg et al. 2001). A Swiss study reported slightly higher prevalences of level 2 (2.2%) and level 3 gambling (0.8%) (Bondolfi et al. 2000). The prevalence of level 3 gambling in Britain fell between these two estimates at 0.7% (Sproston et al. 2000). Furthermore, national research suggests that prevalence rates have remained stable over time. During the mid-1970s, level 3 gambling in the United States was estimated to be 0.7% (Kallick et al. 1979). Twenty years later, two national estimates produced for the National Gambling Impact Study Commission obtained rates of level 3 gambling of 0.9% (National Research Council 1999) and 0.6% (Gerstein et al. 1999).

Understanding level 2 gamblers provides a meaningful opportunity to lower the public health burden associated with gambling disorders. Recent evidence suggests that level 2 gambling is a milder form of pathological gambling (Slutske et al. 2000). Similar to the population-based harms resulting from alcohol use, the majority of such harms resulting from gambling likely are associated with level 2 gambling and not with the most severe cases (Brownson et al. 1997). This circumstance emerges because of the greater number of level 2 gamblers than level 3 or 4 gamblers. Consequently, smaller changes in a larger segment of the population result in a greater impact than larger changes in a smaller population segment. In addition, level 2 gamblers are more responsive to interventions. Efforts to prevent level 2 gamblers from developing clinical disorders represent a useful secondary prevention strategy.

To date, the health care community has taken a medical approach to gambling problems. Although this strategy benefits individuals with severe gambling problems, it makes for a relatively small shift in the social problems that arise from gambling. In addition, an individual approach does little to prevent the development of pathological gambling in other individuals; therefore, the incidence of gambling disorders does not change. A public health perspective would move the focus from the individual to the community and would attempt to shift population gambling norms, thereby reducing the number of level 2 gamblers and improving the health of the population as a whole.

Assessing the Impact of Gambling on the Health of the Public

An integrated public health strategy for understanding gambling requires attention to individuals, populations, and vulnerable population segments. When health problems emerge at the individual level, these difficulties hold the potential to create social impact in the aggregate. That is, problems with very low prevalence rates but very serious consequences can draw population-wide attention (e.g., school massacres, serial sniping). Alternatively, health problems with very high prevalence rates and less dramatic consequences might yield correspondingly widespread attention (e.g., dysthymia among adolescents). The disproportionate distribution of gambling patterns across various population segments has raised concerns about economic, psychological, age-related, and various other potential influences on gambling. These epidemiological observations have evolved into various controversies about the impact of gambling on the public. For example, there is considerable concern about the potential for lottery gambling to be a regressive form of taxation and about whether gambling venues are located disproportionately in low-income areas.

The public policy arena has only recently provided the setting to examine and debate the long-term social, economic, and health impacts arising from the dramatic expansion of gambling (e.g., National Gambling Impact Study Commission 1999). Controversy has surrounded the shifts in the social and political environment that have permitted the growth of gambling. Governments have considerable ambivalence about the appropriate balance between permitting new gambling programs and implementing policies to regulate gambling. The casino industry strenuously lobbies states and municipalities for opportunities to offer its gaming entertainment. Local communities engage in vigorous debate regarding the impact of gambling on the community (e.g., safety and quality of life for neighborhoods and families) (Hornblower 1996). State councils on compulsive or pathological gambling provide public education, help lines, referral services, and advocacy for people and their families affected by gambling-related problems.

Considering Costs and Benefits

A public health position recognizes that gambling has the potential to yield both costs and benefits. These considerations affect all aspects of the community, including health, social, and economic dimensions. A cost-benefit analysis that incorporates the distribution of costs and benefits across a range of subgroups and vulnerable populations is essential to any evaluation of community impact. Only after weighing these matters can a public health strategy be developed that resolves important concerns and supports worthwhile initiatives.

Costs: The Potential Adverse Consequences of Gambling

The scientific literature and the lay media have identified a range of difficulties for individuals, families, and communities that might be related indirectly or directly to gambling (e.g., Ladouceur et al. 1994; Lesieur 1998). These unintended negative consequences can include the following:

1. **Gambling disorders.** The term *gambling disorders* has been used to encompass a spectrum of problems experienced along the continuum that incorporates the constructs of problem and pathological gambling (e.g., Shaffer et al. 1997).
2. **Family dysfunction and domestic violence,** including spousal and child abuse (Bland et al. 1993; Heineman 1989; Jacobs et al. 1989; Lesieur and Rothschild 1989; Lorenz and Yaffee 1988; Moody 1989; Wildman 1989).
3. **Youth and underage gambling** (e.g., Eadington and Cornelius 1993; Shaffer and Hall 1996; Shaffer et al. 1997).
4. **Alcohol and other drug problems** (Crockford and el-Guebaly 1998; Cunningham-Williams et al. 1998; Lesieur and Heineman 1988; Shaffer et al. 1999b; Smart and Ferris 1996; Spunt et al. 1995; Steinberg et al. 1992).
5. **Psychiatric conditions,** including major depression, bipolar disorder, antisocial personality disorder, anxiety, and attention-deficit disorder (e.g., Blaszczynski and Steel 1998; Crockford and el-Guebaly 1998; Cunningham-Williams et al. 1998; Horvath 1998; Knapp and Lech 1987; McCormick et al. 1984; Rugle and Melamed 1993; Shaffer et al. 1999a).
6. **Suicide, suicidal ideation, and suicide attempts** (Bland et al. 1993; Crockford and el-Guebaly 1998; Cunningham-Williams et al. 1998; McCleary et al. 1998; Phillips et al. 1997).
7. **Significant financial problems** as a direct result of wagering, including bankruptcy, loss of employment, and poverty (Blaszczynski and McConaghy 1994; Fessenden 1999; Gerstein et al. 1999; Ladouceur et al. 1994; Lesieur 1998; Marshall 1998).
8. **Criminal behavior,** ranging from prostitution and theft to drug trafficking and homicide (Brown 1987; Gerstein et al. 1999; National Research Council 1999; Smith and Wynne 1999).

Determining whether gambling causes each of these adversities has been—and remains—a knotty and hotly disputed matter. Research suggests that gambling can have a negative impact on health because of associated crime, substance abuse, poverty, and domestic violence (e.g., National Research Council 1999). However, separating cause from effect is difficult. Do criminals gamble, or do gamblers become criminals? Do people with psychological disturbances gamble to treat their emotional circumstance (e.g., Jacobs 1989; Khantzian 1997), or does gambling stimulate these emotional disturbances (e.g., Vaillant 1983)? Like the use of psychoactive substances, these relationships are likely to be related to factors analogous to drug dosage (i.e., the amount of money gambled, the frequency of gambling, and the duration an individual has been en-

gaged in or exposed to gambling). However, as with the positive consequences of gambling, more research is necessary to resolve these important
questions.

The National Research Council and the National Gambling Impact
Study Commission (NGISC) concluded that it was not yet possible to
determine whether gambling caused crime, bankruptcy, domestic violence, or a variety of other perceived adverse social consequences (National Gambling Impact Study Commission 1999; National Research
Council 1999). Some observers had anticipated a different set of findings. Therefore, to ensure the integrity and validity of these conclusions,
the U.S. General Accounting Office (GAO) conducted an independent
review of the evidence and conclusions of NGISC (U.S. General Accounting Office 2000) and added their own research on the Atlantic City
area. The GAO made the following conclusion:

> Neither NGISC nor our Atlantic City case study was able to clearly identify
> the social effects of gambling for a variety of reasons. The amount of high
> quality and relevant research on social effects is extremely limited. While
> data on family problems, crime, and suicide are available, tracking systems
> generally do not collect data on the causes of these incidents, so they cannot
> be linked to gambling. Sometimes data were available only at the county
> level, not for Atlantic City. Further, while studies have shown increases in
> social costs of pathological gamblers, it is difficult to isolate whether gam-
> bling is the only factor causing these problems because pathological gam-
> blers often have other behavior disorders. While NGISC and our case study
> in Atlantic City found some testimonial evidence that gambling, particu-
> larly pathological gambling, has resulted in increased family problems
> (such as domestic violence, child abuse, and divorce), crime, and suicides,
> NGISC reached no conclusions on whether gambling increased family
> problems, crime, or suicide for the general population. Similarly, we found
> no conclusive evidence on whether or not gambling caused increased social
> problems in Atlantic City. (U.S. General Accounting Office 2000, p. 3)

The GAO also failed to find a relationship between gambling and bankrupt-
cies. It can appear that gambling causes social problems, *and it might even be
that gambling is a cause* of these social problems. However, the current state
of scientific research simply does not permit the conclusion that gambling
is the primary or contributing cause of a wide array of social problems (National Research Council 1999; U.S. General Accounting Office 2000).

Benefits: The Potential Positive Health Impacts of Gambling

Most research on gambling has focused on its adverse mental health and
social consequences. To date, with one notable exception (Rosecrance
1988), the study of gambling behavior has ignored the possibility of

health gains associated with gambling. The possibility of "healthy" gambling (Korn and Shaffer 1999; Shaffer and Korn 2002) might help to explain the attraction of gambling. After all, gambling has a negative expected value; therefore, in the absence of alternative explanations, gambling seems to be at odds with people behaving in their self-interest.

Because economic status can affect the emotional, intellectual, physical, and social dimensions of an individual's health (e.g., Evans et al. 1994; Kaplan and Lynch 2001; Wilkinson and Marmot 1998), it follows that gambling can as well. The concept of mental health promotion provides a promising new frame of reference and vocabulary for examining the potential health benefits of gambling. This approach to gambling and health examines the population segments affected by gambling, their mental health promotion goals, and the settings within which these are realized.

The benefits of gambling to mental health promotion can include the following:

1. **Social integration.** Gambling might provide a sense of connectedness and socialization through discretionary leisure-time entertainment. Like going to a movie, being at a pub, or participating in physical activity, going to a casino or a racetrack can provide a healthy change and respite from the demands of everyday life or from social isolation. This activity might be particularly important for older adults.
2. **Adult play** (Smith and Abt 1984). Whereas scientists have long recognized the importance of play for the healthy development of children (Weiss 1995), play might also be particularly important for adults in reducing anxiety, stress, and dysphoria (Ackerman 1999; Driver et al. 1991; Kelly 1982).
3. **Enhancement of coping strategies** by building skills and competencies such as memory enhancement, problem solving through game tactics, mathematical proficiency, concentration, and hand-to-eye physical coordination.

Health benefits can also accrue to communities through gambling-related economic development. Local communities, particularly those with economic problems, can gain significant economic benefits through gambling (National Research Council 1999). Casinos, for example, can act as a community catalyst for economic development. The benefits generally include the creation of jobs in the gambling industry, which in turn stimulates other sectors such as tourism and hospitality. However, observers should interpret projected community health status improvements associated with the expansion of gambling and local economic development with caution, because these economic gains must be sustainable to have a positive health impact. As yet, except for originally impoverished areas, these long-term economic gains for communities have not been demonstrated and currently rest on a complex analysis of projected economic benefit and wealth generation (Nadler 1985; National Gambling Impact Study Commission 1999; National Research Council 1999). Where charity gambling exists (e.g., bingo), gambling-generated monies can go directly to support local nonprofit and charitable organizations in areas such as education, environment, and youth sports. This additional source of revenue can strengthen community capacity by enhancing the health, social service, recreational, and cultural infrastructure. Importantly, gambling generates revenue for state, provincial, and municipal governments, which also can be used to build social capital and reduce reliance on taxation.

Estimating the Costs and Benefits

For communities, groups, and individuals, the central public health question is whether gambling adds to or detracts from the quality of life. Estimates of the health, social, and economic costs of problem and pathological gambling have been proposed, but the methodologies require further refinement (National Research Council 1999). NGISC estimated that the annual cost for problem and pathological gamblers is $5 billion per year and an additional $40 billion in lifetime costs for productivity reduction, social services, and creditor losses. Where casinos have been introduced into a community, it was found that unemployment rates, unemployment insurance, and welfare payments decline by one-seventh and earnings rise in construction, hospitality, transportation, recreation, and amusements sectors (Gerstein et al. 1999). One study suggested that each problem gambler negatively affects 10–17 people, including those in the individual's family and place of employment and those in the government (Politzer et al. 1992). However, taken together, current gambling costs and benefits research rarely highlights the distribution of costs *and* benefits. Consequently, contemporary cost-benefit estimates fail to provide certainty about the nature of this relationship at either the community or the individual level of analysis.

Recommendations for Public Health Policy and Practice

Although limited data support recommendations for public health policy, we suggest the following four steps for public health action (cf. Korn and Shaffer 1999; Shaffer and Korn 2002). First, **adopt strategic goals for gambling;** doing so would provide a focus for public health action and accountability. For example, these goals can include 1) *preventing* gambling-related problems among gamblers in general; 2) *promoting* balanced and informed attitudes, behaviors, and policies toward gambling and gamblers both by individuals and by communities; and 3) *protecting* vulnerable groups from gambling-related harm.

Second, public health workers interested in reducing gambling-related problems should **endorse public health principles.** Three primary principles can guide and inform decision making: 1) ensure that preventing gambling-related problems is a *community priority*, along with the appropriate allocation of resources to primary, secondary, and tertiary prevention initiatives; 2) incorporate a *mental health promotion* approach to gambling, one that builds community capacity, incorporates a holistic view of mental health (including the emotional and spiritual dimensions), and addresses the needs and aspiration of gamblers, individuals at risk for gambling problems, or those affected by them; and 3) foster *personal and social responsibility* for gambling policies and practices.

Third, public health workers who focus on gambling should **incorporate harm-reduction strategies and tactics** (e.g., Tucker et al. 1999). Public health authorities need to embrace harm-reduction strategies directed toward minimizing the adverse health, social, and economic consequences of gambling behavior for individuals, families, and communities. At the very least, these initiatives would include four components: 1) *healthy-gambling guidelines* for the general public (i.e., similar to low-risk-drinking guidelines); 2) vehicles for the *early identification* of gambling problems; 3) *moderation and abstinence goals* for problem gamblers that can be offered nonjudgmentally; and 4) *surveillance and reporting systems* for monitoring gambling-related participation trends as well as the incidence and burden of gambling-related illness.

Finally, a public health strategy would **focus more resources on the identification and treatment of problem and pathological gamblers.** Understanding the behavior of problem gamblers holds considerable potential to lower the social costs and harms associated with gambling disorders.

> The common risk factors for many diseases are present in a large proportion of the population, and therefore, most of the cases of disease arise from the intermediate- and low-risk groups. Relatively small changes in risk among the middle-risk group can result in a greater overall reduction in disease burden than do greater changes in the high-risk group. (Brownson et al. 1997, p. 735)

To illustrate, although pathological gamblers (compared with problem gamblers) represent people with a more intense and potentially destructive relationship with disordered gambling, the former group is considerably smaller. Despite the more moderate and potentially short-lived nature of the problems experienced by problem gamblers, their greater numbers may be responsible for producing more adverse impacts on society. This circumstance is very similar to the observation that problem drinkers are responsible for more aggregate social problems than their alcohol-dependent counterparts (e.g., Sobell and Sobell 1993). As was the case with research on problem drinkers, future gambling research will likely reveal that problem gamblers are more responsive to treatment and social policy interventions than are pathological gamblers. Consequently, a public health strategy that promotes harm reduction and other secondary prevention objectives needs to devote more attention to problem gamblers than is now the case.

Recommendations for Public Health Research

Toward Theory-Guided Research

To advance scientific understanding and the health of the public, new gambling-related research initiatives will require well-developed theoretical maps to guide studies of the distribution and determinants of disordered gambling. For example, no scientific research has established a *causal* link between disordered gambling and either literal or figurative proximity to gambling. Similarly, no scientific research has established a direct link between community cues for gambling and increased urges to gamble—although this is one of the objectives of advertising. Many researchers, however, have noted their concern that a potential link exists between gambling availability and gambling behavior (e.g., Mitka 2001; Pasternak and Fleming 1999; Sibbald 2001; Volberg 2000). Some empirical evidence confirms the importance of this suspicion. For example, a recently published 7-year replication study conducted in Canada showed that in one geographic region, the proportion of local gamblers more than doubled after a local casino opened (Ladouceur et al. 1999). Opening a new casino increased the incidence of people being exposed to gambling. Specifically, before the casino opened, the number of area respondents who gambled was around 14%. After the casino opened, the number of area gamblers reached about 60%. During the same period, individuals from a regional control group without a local casino did not show similar changes in gambling patterns.

Occupation might also contribute to individuals' exposure. If exposure to gambling is the cause of adverse health effects and disordered gambling, then occupational experience with gambling is central to determining its impact. Consistent with this view, casino employees evidence higher prevalence rates of disordered gambling compared with subjects from the general population who are not casino employees (Shaffer and Hall 2002; Shaffer et al. 1999b, 2000).

Exposure

An exposure model implies that the object of addiction causes addictive behavior. Exposure models suggest that the presence of environmental toxins (e.g., gambling settings) increases the likelihood of related disorders (e.g., pathological gambling). Volberg (2002), for example, recently suggested that increasing access to gambling in the United Kingdom would also increase the incidence of problem gamblers: "The number of opportunities to wager in a specified period of time—is tied to the development of gambling problems" (p. 1556). In a recent evaluation of a statewide gambling treatment program in Iowa, an association was found between regional variation in exposure and variation in help seeking for gambling problems; counties more proximate to gambling venues had significantly higher rates of help seeking (Shaffer et al. 2002). An expanded exposure model purports that gamblers' vulnerable or resilient characteristics also play a role in determining the consequences of gambling exposure. For example, exposure to gambling will adversely affect only those who have an underlying vulnerability but not those who are sufficiently resilient (e.g., Jacobs 1989; Khantzian 1975, 1985, 1997).

Adaptation

Alternatively, the social adaptation model suggests that gamblers are dynamic and are capable of changing their behavior in response to exposure (Shaffer and Zinberg 1985; Shaffer et al. 1997; Zinberg 1974, 1975; Zinberg and Fraser 1979; Zinberg and Shaffer 1990). The social adaptation model includes the idea that novelty often stimulates new interest in social activities, but participants eventually adapt to novelty and the effects of these new activities via social learning processes. Therefore, the effects of exposure are limited. For example, adolescents from Nevada were less likely to participate in weekly or more frequent gambling than counterparts in four states with far lower exposure to gambling (Volberg 2001). Furthermore, adolescents from Nevada were less likely to be problem or pathological gamblers than were peers from three of the four other states studied. For many, the process of adaptation can result in unexpected social change. That is, the early increases in new patterns of gambling—whether with or without adverse consequences—are typically followed by an adaptive process that leads to lower levels of involvement or abstinence. Social adaptation can result from decrements in the novelty effect, increases in adverse consequences, the emergence of competing interests, or a combination of these factors—even among some people who evidence fundamental vulnerabilities (e.g., Miller 2000; Shaffer and Jones 1989).

Accuracy of Models

Although individual models of gambling behavior typically lack the scope necessary to shape policy, a public health model has the potential to guide the development of public policy. Every model holds the potential to uniquely influence policy makers and the policies they promulgate. To illustrate, if policy makers subscribe to the exposure model, then they are likely to react very quickly by promulgating regulations designed to control gambling-related problems. However, if the model is accurate, they will have underreacted because the population already is exposed. If the model is incorrect, then they will have overreacted because other forces will emerge to regulate gambling patterns. Conversely, if they subscribe to the adaptation model, then policy makers are likely to react very slowly to changes in patterns of gambling among the population, because they believe that problems will correct themselves.

If the adaptation model is accurate, waiting results in little cost. However, if the adaptation model is incorrect, then regulatory delays risk increased exposure and the incubation of gambling-related harms. The development of a regional index of gambling exposure will allow researchers to evaluate the accuracy of these models and thus inform public policy.

Conclusion

The dramatic expansion of gambling during the latter stages of the twentieth century challenges us to focus on the broad implications for individual and community health. A public health position recognizes that gambling yields both potential costs and benefits. Potential costs or harms associated with gambling include crime, bankruptcy, domestic violence, and gambling disorders. Gambling also benefits society by promoting activities that can enhance mental health and economic development. An integrated public health model is well suited to address matters of healthy public policy, burden of illness, and lifestyle behaviors. Public health efforts should concentrate on specific strategic goals for gambling, endorse public health principles, incorporate harm-reduction strategies and tactics, and focus more resources on the identification and treatment of subclinical gamblers. To help shape future public health efforts, we need a comprehensive research agenda for the gambling field. It is likely that we are now at the end of epidemiological research that focuses only on the general population and at the beginning of a new era of research that features studies of vulnerable populations. This evolution reflects the maturation of a field.

References

Ackerman D: Deep Play. New York, Random House, 1999

American Gaming Association: State of the states: the AGA survey of casino entertainment 2002. Washington, DC, American Gaming Association, 2002. Available at: http://test.americangaming.org/survey/index.cfm. Accessed November 24, 2003.

Bergh C, Eklund T, Sodersten EP: Altered dopamine function in pathological gambling. Psychol Med 27:473–475, 1997

Bland RC, Newman SC, Orn H, et al: Epidemiology of pathological gambling in Edmonton. Can J Psychiatry 38:108–112, 1993

Blaszczynski A, McConaghy N: Criminal offenses in Gamblers Anonymous and hospital treated pathological gamblers. J Gambl Stud 10:99–127, 1994

Blaszczynski A, Steel Z: Personality disorders among pathological gamblers. J Gambl Stud 14:51–71, 1998

Blum K, Braverman ER, Holder MM, et al: Reward deficiency syndrome: a biogenetic model for the diagnosis and treatment of impulsive, addictive, and compulsive behaviors. J Psychoactive Drugs 32 (suppl):i–iv, 1–112, 2000

Bondolfi G, Osiek C, Ferrero F: Prevalence estimates of pathological gambling in Switzerland. Acta Psychiatr Scand 101:473–475, 2000

Breiter HC, Aharon I, Kahneman D, et al: Functional imaging of neural responses to expectancy and experience of monetary gains and losses. Neuron 30:619–639, 2001

Brown RIF: Pathological gambling and associated patterns of crime: comparisons with alcohol and other drug addictions. Journal of Gambling Behavior 3:98–114, 1987

Brownson RC, Newschaffer CJ, Ali-Abarghoui F: Policy research for disease prevention: challenges and practical recommendations. Am J Public Health 87:735–739, 1997

Christiansen EM: Gambling and the American economy, in Gambling: Socioeconomic Impacts and Public Policy. Edited by Frey JH. Thousand Oaks, CA, Sage, 1998, pp 36–52

Comings DE: The molecular genetics of pathological gambling. CNS Spectr 3:20–37, 1998

Crockford DN, el-Guebaly N: Psychiatric comorbidity in pathological gambling: a critical review. Can J Psychiatry 43:43–50, 1998

Cunningham-Williams RM, Cottler LB, Compton WM III, et al: Taking chances: problem gamblers and mental health disorders—results from the St. Louis Epidemiologic Catchment Area Study. Am J Public Health 88:1093–1096, 1998

Driver BL, Brown PJ, Peterson GL (eds): Benefits of Leisure. State College, PA, Venture Publishing, 1991

Eadington WR, Cornelius JA (eds): Gambling Behavior and Problem Gambling. Reno, NV, Institute for the Study of Gambling and Commercial Gaming, College of Business Administration, University of Nevada, Reno, 1993

Evans RG, Barer ML, Marmor TR (eds): Why Are Some People Healthy and Others Not? The Determinants of Health of Populations. New York, Aldine de Gruyter, 1994

Fessenden F: Lottery cost is heaviest on the poor. New York Times, May 22, 1999, p A12

Freud S: Dostoevsky and parricide (1928), in The Standard Edition of the Complete Psychological Works of Sigmund Freud, Vol 21. Translated and edited by Strachey J. London, Hogarth Press, 1961, pp 175–196

Gerstein D, Murphy S, Toce M, et al: Gambling Impact and Behavior Study: Report to the National Gambling Impact Study Commission. Chicago, IL, National Opinion Research Center, 1999

Heineman M: Parents of male compulsive gamblers: clinical issues/treatment approaches. Journal of Gambling Behavior 5:321–333, 1989

Hollander E, Buchalter AJ, DeCaria CM: Pathological gambling. Psychiatr Clin N Am 23:629–642, 2000

Hornblower M: No dice: the backlash against gambling. Time, April 1, 1996, pp 29–33

Horvath TA: Sex, Drugs, Gambling, and Chocolate: A Workbook for Overcoming Addictions. San Luis Obispo, CA, Impact, 1998

Jacobs DF: A general theory of addictions: rationale for and evidence supporting a new approach for understanding and treating addictive behaviors, in Compulsive Gambling: Theory, Research and Practice. Edited by Shaffer HJ, Stein S, Gambino B, et al. Lexington, MA, Lexington Books, 1989, pp 35–64

Jacobs DF, Marston AR, Singer RD, et al: Children of problem gamblers. Journal of Gambling Behavior 5:261–267, 1989

Kallick M, Suits D, Dielman T, et al: A Survey of American Gambling Attitudes and Behavior (Research Report Series). Ann Arbor, MI, Survey Research Center, Institute for Social Research, University of Michigan, 1979

Kaplan GA, Lynch JW: Is economic policy health policy? Am J Public Health 91:351–353, 2001

Kelly J: Leisure. Englewood Cliffs, NJ, Prentice-Hall, 1982

Khantzian EJ: Self selection and progression in drug dependence. Psychiatry Dig 36:19–22, 1975

Khantzian EJ: The self-medication hypothesis of addictive disorders: focus on heroin and cocaine dependence. Am J Psychiatry 142:1259–1264, 1985

Khantzian EJ: The self-medication hypothesis of substance use disorders: a reconsideration and recent applications. Harv Rev Psychiatry 4:231–244, 1997

Knapp TJ, Lech BC: Pathological gambling: a review with recommendations. Advances in Behavioral Research and Therapy 9:21–49, 1987

Korn DA, Shaffer HJ: Gambling and the health of the public: adopting a public health perspective. J Gambl Stud 15:289–365, 1999

Ladouceur R, Boisvert JM, Pepin M, et al: Social costs of pathological gambling. J Gambl Stud 10:399–409, 1994

Ladouceur R, Jacques C, Ferland F, et al: Prevalence of problem gambling: a replication study 7 years later. Can J Psychiatry 44:802–804, 1999

Lesieur HR: Costs and treatment of pathological gambling. Ann Am Acad Pol Soc Sci 556:153–171, 1998

Lesieur HR, Heineman M: Pathological gambling among youthful multiple substance abusers in a therapeutic community. Br J Addict 83:765–771, 1988

Lesieur HR, Rothschild J: Children of Gamblers Anonymous members. Journal of Gambling Behavior 5:269–281, 1989

Lindner RM: The psychodynamics of gambling. Ann Am Acad Pol Soc Sci 269:93–107, 1950

Lorenz VC, Yaffee R: Pathological gambling: psychosomatic, emotional and marital difficulties as reported by the spouse. Journal of Gambling Behavior 4:13–26, 1988

Marshall K: The gambling industry: raising the stakes. Perspectives on Labour and Income 10:7–11, 1998

McCleary R, Chew K, Feng W, et al: Suicide and Gambling: An Analysis of Suicide Rates in U.S. Counties and Metropolitan Areas (Prepared for the American Gaming Association). Irvine CA, School of Social Ecology, University of California–Irvine, 1998

McCormick RA, Russo AM, Ramirez LF, et al: Affective disorders among pathological gamblers seeking treatment. Am J Psychiatry 141:215–218, 1984

Miller WR: Rediscovering fire: small interventions, large effects. Psychol Addict Behav 14:6–18, 2000

Mitka M: Win or lose, Internet gambling stakes are high. JAMA 285:1005, 2001

Moody G: Parents of young gamblers. Journal of Gambling Behavior 5:313–320, 1989

Nadler LB: The epidemiology of pathological gambling: critique of existing research and alternative strategies. Journal of Gambling Behavior 1:35–50, 1985

National Gambling Impact Study Commission: National Gambling Impact Study Commission Final Report. Washington, DC, National Gambling Impact Study Commission, 1999. Available at: http://govinfo.library.unt.edu/ngisc/reports/fullrpt.html. Accessed November 28, 2003.

National Research Council: Pathological Gambling: A Critical Review. Washington, DC, National Academy Press, 1999

Pasternak AV, Fleming MF: Prevalence of gambling disorders in a primary care setting. Arch Fam Med 8:515–520, 1999

Phillips DP, Welty WR, Smith MM: Elevated suicide levels associated with legalized gambling. Suicide Life Threat Behav 27:373–378, 1997

Politzer RM, Yesalis CE, Hudak CJ: The epidemiologic model and the risk of legalized gambling: where are we headed? Health Values 16:20–27, 1992

Quinn JP: Fools of Fortune; or, Gambling and Gamblers. Chicago, IL, Anti-Gambling Association, 1892

Rosecrance J: Gambling Without Guilt: The Legitimation of an American Pastime. Pacific Grove, CA, Brooks/Cole, 1988

Rugle L, Melamed L: Neuropsychological assessment of attention problems in pathological gamblers. J Nerv Ment Dis 181:107–112, 1993

Shaffer HJ, Hall MN: Estimating the prevalence of adolescent gambling disorders: a quantitative synthesis and guide toward standard gambling nomenclature. J Gambl Stud 12:193–214, 1996

Shaffer HJ, Hall MN: Updating and refining prevalence estimates of disordered gambling behaviour in the United States and Canada. Can J Public Health 92:168–172, 2001

Shaffer HJ, Hall MN: Longitudinal patterns of gambling and drinking problems among casino employees. J Soc Psychol 142:405–424, 2002

Shaffer HJ, Jones SB: Quitting Cocaine: The Struggle Against Impulse. Lexington, MA, Lexington Books, 1989

Shaffer HJ, Kidman R: Shifting perspectives on gambling and addiction. J Gambl Stud 19:1–6, 2003

Shaffer HJ, Korn DA: Gambling and related mental disorders: a public health analysis. Annu Rev Public Health 23:171–212, 2002

Shaffer HJ, Zinberg NE: The social psychology of intoxicant use: the natural history of social settings and social control. Bulletin of the Society of Psychologists in the Addictive Behaviors 4:49–55, 1985

Shaffer HJ, Hall MN, Vander Bilt J: Estimating the Prevalence of Disordered Gambling Behavior in the United States and Canada: A Meta-Analysis. Boston, MA, Harvard Medical School, Division on Addictions, 1997

Shaffer HJ, Hall MN, Vander Bilt J: Estimating the prevalence of disordered gambling behavior in the United States and Canada: a research synthesis. Am J Public Health 89:1369–1376, 1999a

Shaffer HJ, Vander Bilt J, Hall MN: Gambling, drinking, smoking and other health risk activities among casino employees. Am J Ind Med 36:365–378, 1999b

Shaffer HJ, Eber G, Hall MN, et al: Smoking behavior among casino employees: self-report validation using plasma cotinine. Addict Behav 25:693–704, 2000

Shaffer HJ, LaBrie RA, LaPlante DA, et al: The Iowa Department of Public Health Gambling Treatment Services: Four Years of Evidence (Technical Report No 101102-200). Boston, MA, Harvard Medical School, 2002

Sibbald B: Casinos bring ill fortune, psychiatrists warn. CMAJ 164:388, 2001

Skinner HA: Gambling: achieving the right balance. J Gambl Stud 15:285–287, 1999

Slutske WS, Eisen S, True WR, et al: Common genetic vulnerability for pathological gambling and alcohol dependence in men. Arch Gen Psychiatry 57:666–673, 2000

Smart RG, Ferris J: Alcohol, drugs and gambling in the Ontario adult population, 1994. Can J Psychiatry 41:36–45, 1996

Smith GJ, Wynne HJ: Gambling and Crime in Western Canada: Exploring Myth and Reality. Calgary, AB, Canada West Foundation, 1999

Smith JF, Abt V: Gambling as play. Ann Am Acad Pol Soc Sci 474:122–132, 1984

Sobell MB, Sobell LC: Treatment for problem drinkers: a public health priority, in Addictive Behaviors Across the Life Span: Prevention, Treatment, and Policy Issues. Edited by Baer JS, Marlatt GA, McMahon RJ. Newbury Park, CA, Sage, 1993, pp 138–157

Sproston K, Erens B, Orford J: Gambling Behaviour in Britain: Results From the British Gambling Prevalence Survey. London, National Centre for Social Research, 2000

Spunt B, Lesieur H, Hunt D, et al: Gambling among methadone patients. Int J Addict 30:929–962, 1995

Steinberg M, Kosten T, Rounsaville B: Cocaine abuse and pathological gambling. Am J Addict 1:121–132, 1992

Tucker JA, Donovan DM, Marlatt GA (eds): Changing Addictive Behavior. New York, Guilford, 1999

U.S. General Accounting Office: Impact of Gambling: Economic Effects More Measurable Than Social Effects. Report to the Honorable Frank R. Wolf, House of Representatives (GAO/GGD-00-78). Washington, DC, U.S. General Accounting Office, 2000

Vaillant GE: The Natural History of Alcoholism: Causes, Patterns, and Paths to Recovery. Cambridge, MA, Harvard University Press, 1983

Volberg RA: The future of gambling in the United Kingdom: increasing access creates more problem gamblers (editorial). BMJ 320:1556, 2000

Volberg RA: Gambling and problem gambling among adolescents in Nevada. Nevada Department of Human Resources, 2001. Available at: http://www.geminiresearch.com (click on Reports and Links). Accessed May 13, 2002.

Volberg RA, Abbott MW, Rönnberg S, et al: Prevalence and risks of pathological gambling in Sweden. Acta Psychiatr Scand 104:250–256, 2001

Weiss MR: Children in sport: an educational model, in Sport Psychology Interventions. Edited by Murphy SM. Champaign, IL, Human Kinetics, 1995, pp 39–70

Wildman RW: Pathological gambling: marital-familial factors, implications, and treatments. Journal of Gambling Behavior 5:293–301, 1989

Wilkinson R, Marmot M (eds): Social Determinants of Health: The Solid Facts. Copenhagen, World Health Organization Regional Office for Europe, 1998

Zinberg NE: High States: A Beginning Study (Publ No SS-3). Washington, DC, Drug Abuse Council, 1974

Zinberg NE: Addiction and ego function. Psychoanal Study Child 30:567–588, 1975

Zinberg NE, Fraser KM: The role of the social setting in the prevention and treatment of alcoholism, in The Diagnosis and Treatment of Alcoholism. Edited by Mendelson J, Mello N. New York, McGraw-Hill, 1979, pp 359–385

Zinberg NE, Shaffer HJ: Essential factors of a rational policy on intoxicant use. J Drug Issues 20:619–627, 1990

Epidemiology

Renee M. Cunningham-Williams, Ph.D., M.P.E.
Linda B. Cottler, Ph.D.
Sharon B. Womack, Ph.D., M.P.E.

One of the first steps in understanding a social, behavioral, or health disorder is to examine how widespread it is and—in terms of key socio-demographic factors—who is affected by it. Epidemiology is a field of study that attempts to determine the prevalence of a disorder and the number of new cases that appear in a given time period (i.e., incidence). Since 1975, there have been four major efforts to estimate the prevalences of gambling activity and pathological gambling in the United States. Three of these studies, as well as several site-specific studies, were recently reviewed (Cunningham-Williams and Cottler 2001). The first national study of gambling attitudes, published before the inclusion of pathological gambling in DSM-III (American Psychiatric Association 1980), was the result of the findings of a United States presidential commission, the Commission on the Review of the National Policy Toward Gambling (Kallick et al. 1979). Using the term *compulsive gambling*, this study reported lifetime rates for "probable compulsive gambling" of 0.8% and for a less severe form of problem gambling, "potential compulsive gambling," of 2.3%. This study was important because it drew national research attention to gambling activity for the first time in America and provided national estimates of problem gambling. In addition, it showed that although more than half of Americans reported some form of gambling annually—including social betting among friends, purchasing lottery tickets, and pari-mutuel wagering—heavy betting was more often reported by males, nonwhites, and persons with higher socioeconomic status (Kallick et al. 1979; Welte et al. 2002).

It was not until two decades later that another national study, a United States presidential commission report from the National Gambling Impact Study Commission, was published. This study—the first of its kind since the inclusion of pathological gambling as a psychiatric disorder in DSM-III—was conducted by the National Opinion Research Center (1999). It included an adult telephone survey ($n=2,417$) and a survey of gambling patrons ($n=530$) (Gerstein et al. 1999). Estimates of lifetime (0.8%) and past-year pathological gambling (0.1%) were presented based on the telephone survey. These estimates increased slightly when the additional gambling patrons were included in the analysis (lifetime, 1.2%; past year, 0.6%). Unfortunately, the patron portion of this publicly accessible data set may have limited utility because of the low response rates at some of the interview sites and the questionable validity of the patron data (Gambling Impact and Behavior Study 2001).

Using random-digit dialing methodology, investigators at the Research Institute on Addictions (Welte et al. 2002) conducted a study among a representative sample of adults age 18 years and older. The researchers found a gambling participation rate of 82% (about 20% higher than the two earlier national studies), with lottery and casino gambling having the highest participation rates. The significantly higher participation reported in this study is likely due to differences in sampling strategies and assessments used across the studies (Welte et al. 2002). Using weighted percentages analyzed from scores on the DSM-IV Diagnostic Interview Schedule (Version 4.0) (Robins et al. 1997), the researchers found for all respondents a lifetime pathological gambling rate (i.e., five or more criteria satisfied) of 2.0% and a past-year pathological gambling rate of 1.35% (Welte et al. 2002; J.W. Welte, personal communication, April 21, 2003). The conditional prevalence estimates (i.e., the estimates among the 92.8% of those who had gambled at some time in their lives) of pathological gambling were slightly higher (lifetime, 2.16%; past year, 1.46%). For the 82.2% of respondents who had gambled in the past year, the lifetime rate was 2.4%, and the past-year rate was 1.64%. For problem gambling (i.e., three or four criteria met), the entire sample had a lifetime rate of 2.77% and a past-year rate of 2.17%; among gamblers only, the lifetime rate was 2.98% and the past-year rate was 2.34%; and among those who had gambled in the past year, the lifetime rate was 3.19% and the past-year rate was 2.57%.

These estimates are similar to those compiled by a committee of the National Research Council (1999). This committee conducted a reanalysis of 49 general-population studies from Shaffer and Hall's (1997) meta-analysis of 120 United States and Canadian studies published between 1975 and 1997. The pathological gambling rates from the meta-analysis were 1.5% (lifetime) and 0.9% (past year). As with other studies, the problem gambling rate was at least two to three times as high as the pathological gambling estimates (lifetime, 5.4%; past year, 2.9%).

Studies conducted in certain geographic regions mirror, to a large extent, the national estimates. One such study, the St. Louis Epidemiologic Catchment Area (ECA) household survey ($N=3,004$), conducted in 1981 (Robins et al. 1981), found a lifetime pathological gambling rate of 0.9% and a problem gambling rate of 9.2% (Cunningham-Williams et al. 1998). The St. Louis, Missouri, site was one of five participating sites in the ECA study and was the only site to include pathological gambling among the mental disorders assessed. The analysis of pathological gambling at the St. Louis site is the first and only household study in the United States to report prevalence estimates of problem gambling and of DSM-III pathological gambling. The St. Louis survey also has the only known incidence data (i.e., the number of new cases of a disorder among a population that was interviewed at an earlier point in time) collected from household residents in the United States (Cottler and Cunningham-Williams 1998). Using a subsample of ECA study participants ($n=162$), persons who were drug users at baseline and who were reinterviewed 11 years later, we found that the number of nongamblers decreased (from 93 to 73) and that the pathological gambling incidence rate increased from 1.2% (2 of 162) to 3.7% (6 of 162). A more striking increase was found for problem gambling (an increase from 3.7% to 10.5%).

More recently, in a five-state study of problem gambling using the South Oaks Gambling Screen (SOGS) (see Appendix D), Volberg (1994) found rates of "probable pathological gambling" of 0.1% (in Iowa) to 2.3% (in Maryland). Another site-specific study among adults in Oregon ($n=1,502$) reported a lifetime probable pathological gambling rate of 1.8% (past year, 1.4%) and a lifetime problem gambling rate of 3.1% (past year, 1.9%) (Volberg 1997). Estimates obtained using the SOGS for Louisiana adults age 21 years and older were 3.0% for problem gambling and 1.4% for probable pathological gambling (Westphal and Rush 1996).

Problem and pathological gambling are international phenomena. Adult rates similar to those found in the United States and Canada are found in New Zealand (Abbott 2001), Sweden (Volberg et al. 2001), Britain (Sproston et al. 2000), Hong Kong (Centre for Social Policy Studies 2002), Australia (Productivity Commission 1999), South Africa (Collins and Barr 2001), and Switzerland (Bondolfi et al. 2000). These studies used the SOGS and/or DSM-IV (American Psychiatric Association 1994) pathological gambling assessments and reported rates averaging about 1% for probable pathological gambling, with the highest rates being found in Hong Kong (1.9%) ("Disordered Gambling" 2002).

Sociodemographic Correlates

An important consideration of epidemiology is how disease affects various population groups. Most investigations have reported that men are more often involved in gambling activity and have higher rates of problem gambling and pathological gambling. Most early studies took samples from settings in which men were overrepresented (e.g., Gamblers Anonymous, Veterans Administration hospitals, or drug treatment settings) (Cunningham-Williams and Cottler 2001). Nevertheless, recent observations tend to concur that men have rates of pathological gambling that are twice as high as those of women (Cunningham-Williams et al. 1998; National Research Council 1999; Volberg 1994; Welte et al. 2002).

With respect to age, there does not yet appear to be evidence supporting higher pathological gambling rates in middle-aged and older populations (National Research Council 1999). Older populations may be vulnerable to gambling problems because of more disposable time and income (McNeilly and Burke 2001) associated with retirement and other life changes. Yet there is a suggestion that we may be presuming that this population is vulnerable and fail to recognize that there are social benefits to their gambling behaviors (Hope and Havir 2002; Laundergan et al. 1990). More complete discussions of public health and aspects of gambling behaviors among older adults are found in Chapter 1, "Gambling and the Public Health," and Chapter 6, "Older Adults."

A national longitudinal study of pathological gambling among children, adolescents, and young adults has not yet been conducted. However, site-specific investigations have found similarly high rates of problem gambling and pathological gambling among adolescents (see Chapter 5, "Adolescents and Young Adults," and Chapter 11, "Prevention and Treatment of Adolescent Problem and Pathological Gambling").

There is a dearth of research reporting rates specific to certain population groups—particularly various racial and ethnic groups and groups of varying socioeconomic profiles—using representative samples. Even fewer studies have disentangled race and ethnicity from social class in reporting prevalence rates (Cunningham-Williams and Cottler 2001; National Research Council 1999). Nevertheless, available evidence suggests that in the United States, pathological gambling is most prevalent among racial and ethnic minority populations and among those of lower socio-economic classes. The ECA study (Cunningham-Williams et al. 1998) found that twice as many African Americans were problem gamblers (31%) than were nonproblem gamblers (15%). High rates of pathological gambling have also been reported for African American adults (Volberg 1994; Volberg and Abbott 1997), African American adolescents (Stinch-field et al. 1997), Latin American adolescents (Stinchfield et al. 1997), Asians (Zane and Huh-Kim 1998), and Aboriginal populations (Stinch-field et al. 1997; Volberg 1997; Zitzow 1996; see review of Aboriginal studies in Wardman et al. 2001).

The majority of studies have been conducted among treated popula-tions with high rates of comorbidity (ranging from 7% to 16%), and these studies have been extensively reviewed elsewhere (National Research Council 1999). It is important to note that high rates of psychiatric and substance use disorder comorbidity—particularly for nicotine depen-dence, alcohol abuse and dependence, depression, and antisocial person-ality disorder—have been found in studies of the general population (Cunningham-Williams et al. 1998), studies of adult drug users both in and out of treatment (Cunningham-Williams et al. 2000; Hall et al. 2000), studies of adolescent outpatients (Petry and Tawfik 2001), and studies of homeless persons seeking treatment for substance use disorders (Shaffer et al. 2002).

Internet Gambling: An Emerging Trend

The opportunities to participate in gambling behaviors have increased considerably, with the advent of computers and new technologies mak-ing Internet access readily available to users in their homes, their offices, and other locations. As a result, people can participate in gambling activ-ities not only at the local casino but at home or anywhere and at any time. Reportedly, 66% of all adults (52% female, 76% Caucasian) in the United States are Internet users, with 55% accessing the Internet from home and 30% accessing online gambling opportunities in the workplace (Taylor 2002).

According to the Ipsos Reid Group (2000), 85% of Americans ages 12–24 years use the Internet regularly. By 2005, more than 40 million U.S. children under age 18 are expected to be online (Grunwald Associ-ates 2000). This rapidly growing group of Internet users raises questions regarding adolescents' exposure to and vulnerability for gambling prob-lems (Griffiths and Wood 2000).

Worldwide, electronic gambling is one of the hottest sectors on the Internet (Gareiss and Soat 2002). Indeed, Internet gambling is growing at a dramatic rate. In 1998, more than 600 online gambling sites existed (Kirkman 1998), and by 2000 this number had grown to over 800 (Turner 2002). According to the National Gambling Impact Study Commission (1999), by 1998 the number of Internet gamblers had grown to 14.5 million, producing $651 million in revenue. Furthermore, electronic gambling revenue has been projected to grow from nearly $3 billion via the Internet in 2002 to around $8 billion in 2006 (Gareiss and Soat 2002).

The first Native American lottery on the Internet, US Lottery, was established by the Coeur d'Alene tribe in 1997 (Rose 2000). Subsequently, other tribes have opened online bingo and casino sites. Although Native American tribes have been able to legally use the Internet for gambling operations (Kirkman 1998), it was not until June 2001 that Nevada became the first state in the United States to legalize online gambling (Wharry 2001). According to current projections, it is anticipated that online gambling revenue will double Nevada's reported 2001 earnings of approximately $4.56 billion in 2003 (Wharry 2001). However, legal issues surrounding Internet gambling remain to be resolved. Indeed, legislation concerning issues related to the legality of Internet gambling in the United States is being addressed by several states.

The Internet is a relatively new technology that provides gambling access and therefore is an important consideration in studies of pathological gambling. Important issues related to pathological gambling concern the ease of access, anonymity, interactivity, convenience, isolation, and asocial nature of online gaming activities (Griffiths and Parke 2002; Wharry 2001). One finding noted in a small qualitative study of Internet and non-Internet gamblers was that Internet gamblers cited convenience and tax-free betting as being related to their desire to gamble on the Internet (Parke and Griffiths 2001). In addition, Internet and non-Internet gamblers differed on issues related to financial stability, competitiveness, motivation, physiological effects, and social facilitation (Griffiths and Parke 2002).

Preliminary findings from the St. Louis Area Personality, Health and Lifestyle Survey 2001 (N=914), obtained using the Internet/Computer Assessment Module (Womack et al. 2001) and the self-administered DSM-IV Gambling Assessment Module (Cunningham-Williams et al. 2001), indicate that 90% of the sample reported using a computer, with 83% of them using the Internet. Among Internet users, 3.2% reported using the Internet as a means to gamble (Womack et al. 2002). Although no gender differences were apparent in this preliminary study, Internet gamblers compared with non-Internet gamblers were younger and were more likely to report going to other venues to gamble more than five times in their lifetime (88% vs. 59%).

Results of the first United Kingdom Internet study ($N=2,098$) showed a 24% rate of Internet use, with a conditional prevalence rate of Internet gambling among Internet users of 1% (Griffiths 2002). Furthermore, women reported that Internet gambling was safer (2%), less intimidating (9%), anonymous (9%), more fun (2%), and more tempting (13%). However, no evidence was found of problem gambling behaviors associated with Internet gambling in that sample.

Much lower rates of Internet use during the past 12 months were found in a Canadian study ($N=1,294$) (Ialomiteanu and Adlaf 2001), in which rates among women (6.3%) were higher than among men (4.9%). Only marital status was significantly related to Internet gambling, with those divorced or widowed being more likely to gamble online compared with those who were married (10.9% vs. 4.9%). In addition, among gamblers reporting past-year gambling, 6.7% reported Internet gambling, with those age 65 years and older reporting the highest rates of Internet gambling.

Some research suggests that Internet gamblers may have more serious gambling problems than those who gamble at other venues. According to Ladd and Petry (2002), of the 8.1% of their respondents who reported lifetime gambling on the Internet, 3.7% reported gambling on the Internet at least weekly. The combined lifetime rate for problem and more severe gambling was 26%, with 74% of those who gambled on the Internet being classified as problem or pathological gamblers. Surprisingly, lower education and income levels were reported by Internet gamblers compared with non-Internet gamblers in this study. Although age and ethnicity differences were found between those with and without Internet gambling experience, no gender differences were found.

Thus, with the addition of the Internet as an emerging technology in the field of gambling, it is expected that greater attention will be paid to its contribution to rates of pathological gambling and varying typologies of gamblers in the years to come. Learning how to determine the demographic characteristics of Internet gamblers without invading their privacy is a challenge but is one that must be taken.

Assessment Development in Pathological Gambling Research

Given the changing DSM criteria for pathological gambling, it is not surprising that assessments of pathological gambling vary in their concordance with current diagnostic criteria. There are two major classifications of assessments: screening and diagnostic. Screening assessments are used to determine the probability that a disorder is present in a group of apparently well persons, so that those with a high probability can be administered further diagnostic testing. Diagnostic assessments cover the full range of criteria needed to formulate an actual diagnosis of the disorder. Assessments can be structured or semistructured and can be administered by a clinician, a trained nonclinician (lay) interviewer, or a computer, or they can be self-administered.

Other concerns in developing assessments center on the establishment of various psychometric properties, namely, reliability and validity. Reliability is a measure of consistency of two raters or two instruments. It addresses whether consistent measurement of the same phenomenon was achieved—in the same way, at each and every measurement occasion, across various settings, and across various interviewers (or raters). Validity is generally concerned with the notions of accuracy and precision. In other words, it answers the question, "Am I accurately and precisely measuring what I intend to measure?"

Furthermore, a particular challenge in the development of assessment tools is establishing construct validity. Construct validity is the degree to which an instrument accurately taps the underlying theoretical construct on which it is based (Corcoran and Fisher 2000) and is determined in part by whether it correlates with other similar assessments of the same construct. Central to establishing construct validity is the development of appropriate assessment tools that are designed to measure the underlying construct being investigated, a process that ultimately affects prevalence estimates. Chapter 14, "Screening and Assessment Instruments," provides a detailed discussion of specific instruments.

Conclusion

In this chapter, we presented a summary of problem gambling and pathological gambling prevalence estimates derived from several national and site-specific studies and discussed how the Internet may change the prevalence of pathological gambling. There is a distinct need for incidence and longitudinal data to elucidate the course of the disorder. The understanding of the epidemiology of pathological gambling is hampered by the relative lack of investigations involving general-population samples and by limited stratification of important sociodemographic groups, including those defined by race or ethnicity and by social class. In addition, estimates of the prevalence of pathological gambling may be underreported or overreported, depending on the sample.

As a form of entertainment, gambling is widespread. Although rates of pathological gambling among gamblers are low, the impact of the disorder is high. So that clinicians can better address the problem with patients affected by pathological gambling, as much as possible should be learned about who is affected by gambling, the subtypes of the disorder, and its duration and progression. To provide effective policies, prevention, and treatment, a greater understanding of the epidemiology of pathological gambling must be gained. Therefore, researchers need to identify and address nosological and methodological issues that challenge current understanding.

References

Abbott MW: Problem and Non-Problem Gamblers in New Zealand: A Report on Phase Two of the 1999 National Prevalence Survey. Wellington, New Zealand Department of Internal Affairs, 2001

American Psychiatric Association: Diagnostic and Statistical Manual of Mental Disorders, 3rd Edition. Washington, DC, American Psychiatric Association, 1980

American Psychiatric Association: Diagnostic and Statistical Manual of Mental Disorders, 4th Edition. Washington, DC, American Psychiatric Association, 1994

Bondolfi G, Osiek C, Ferrero F: Prevalence estimates of pathological gambling in Switzerland. Acta Psychiatr Scand 101:473–475, 2000

Centre for Social Policy Studies: Report on a Study of Hong Kong People's Participation in Gambling Activities. Hong Kong, Department of Applied Social Sciences and General Education Centre of the Hong Kong Polytechnic University, 2002

Collins P, Barr G: Gambling and Problem Gambling in South Africa: A National Study. Cape Town, National Centre for the Study of Gambling, 2001

Corcoran K, Fisher J: Measures for Clinical Practice: A Sourcebook, 3rd Edition. New York, Free Press, 2000

Cottler LB, Cunningham-Williams RM: The 11 year incidence of gambling problems among drug users recruited from the St. Louis ECA study. Paper presented to the National Academy of Sciences Workshop on the Social and Economic Impact of Gambling, Washington, DC, June 1–3, 1998

Cunningham-Williams RM, Cottler LB: The epidemiology of pathological gambling. Semin Clin Neuropsychiatry 6:155–166, 2001

Cunningham-Williams RM, Cottler LB, Compton WM III, et al: Taking chances: problem gamblers and mental health disorders—results from the St. Louis Epidemiologic Catchment Area Study. Am J Public Health 88:1093–1096, 1998

Cunningham-Williams RM, Cottler LB, Compton WM, et al: Problem gambling and comorbid psychiatric and substance use disorders among drug users recruited from drug treatment and community settings. J Gambl Stud 16:347–376, 2000

Cunningham-Williams RM, Cottler LB, Books S, et al: Gambling Assessment Module IV, Short Form, Self-Administered (GAM-IV-S). St. Louis, MO, Washington University, 2001

Disordered gambling as an international phenomenon. WAGER (Weekly Addiction Gambling Education Report) 7(51), 2002. Available at: http://www.thewager.org/backissues.htm. Accessed November 29, 2003.

Gambling Impact and Behavior Study: part 3. WAGER (Weekly Addiction Gambling Education Report) 6(32), 2001. Available at: http://www.thewager.org/backissues.htm. Accessed November 29, 2003.

Gareiss R, Soat J: Let it ride: sure, gambling seems like a perfect business model for the Web. But is it legal? Information Week, July 8, 2002, pp 59–66

Gerstein D, Murphy S, Toce M, et al: Gambling Impact and Behavior Study: Final Report to the National Gambling Impact Study Commission. Chicago, IL, National Opinion Research Center, 1999

Griffiths M: Internet gambling: preliminary results of the first U.K. prevalence study. Electronic Journal of Gambling Issues (5), 2002. Available at: http://www.camh.net/egambling/issue5/research/griffiths_article.html. Accessed November 27, 2003.

Griffiths M, Parke J: The social impact of Internet gambling. Soc Sci Comput Rev 20:312–320, 2002

Griffiths M, Wood RT: Risk factors in adolescence: the case of gambling, video-game playing, and the Internet. J Gambl Stud 16:199–225, 2000

Grunwald Associates: Children, Families, and the Internet. San Mateo, CA, Grunwald Associates, 2000. Available at: http://www.grunwald.com/survey/newsrelease.html. Accessed November 29, 2003.

Hall GW, Carriero NJ, Takushi RY, et al: Pathological gambling among cocaine-dependent outpatients. Am J Psychiatry 157:1127–1133, 2000

Hope J, Havir L: You bet they're having fun! Older Americans and casino gambling. J Aging Stud 16:177–197, 2002

Ialomiteanu A, Adlaf E: Internet gambling among Ontario adults. Electronic Journal of Gambling Issues (5), 2001. Available at: http://www.camh.net/egambling/issue5/research/ialomiteanu_adlaf_article.html. Accessed November 27, 2003.

Ipsos Reid Group: American youth global Internet pacesetters. New York, Ipsos North America, 2000. Available at: http://www.ipsos-pa.com/dsp_displaypr_us.cfm?id_to_view=1025. Accessed November 29, 2003.

Kallick MD, Suits T, Deilman T, et al: A Survey of American Gambling Attitudes and Behavior (Research Report Series, Survey Research Center, Institute for Social Research). Ann Arbor, MI, University of Michigan Press, 1979

Kirkman CS: Gambling on the Internet. Web Techniques, March 1998. Available at: http://www.webtechniques.com/archives/1998/03/just/. Accessed November 27, 2003.

Ladd GT, Petry NM: Disordered gambling among university-based medical and dental patients: a focus on Internet gambling. Psychol Addict Behav 16:76–79, 2002

Laundergan JC, Schaefer J, Eckhoff K, et al: Adult Survey of Minnesota Gambling Behavior: A Benchmark. St. Paul, MN, Minnesota Department of Human Services, Mental Health Division, 1990

McNeilly DP, Burke WJ: Gambling as a social activity of older adults. Int J Aging Hum Dev 52:19–28, 2001

National Gambling Impact Study Commission: National Gambling Impact Study Commission Final Report. Washington, DC, National Gambling Impact Study Commission, 1999. Available at: http://govinfo.library.unt.edu/ngisc/reports/fullrpt.html. Accessed November 28, 2003.

National Opinion Research Center: Gambling Impact and Behavior Study: Report to the National Gambling Impact Study Commission. Chicago, IL, National Opinion Research Center at the University of Chicago, 1999. Available at: http://www.norc.uchicago.edu/new/gamb-fin.htm. Accessed December 13, 2003.

National Research Council: Pathological Gambling: A Critical Review. Washington, DC, National Academy Press, 1999

Parke J, Griffiths MD: Internet gambling: a small qualitative pilot study. Results from "Betting the Couch." Paper presented at the Psychology and the Internet Conference, British Psychological Society, Farnborough, UK, November 7–9, 2001

Petry NM, Tawfik Z: Comparison of problem-gambling and non-problem-gambling youths seeking treatment for marijuana abuse. J Am Acad Child Adolesc Psychiatry 40:1324–1331, 2001

Productivity Commission: Australia's Gambling Industries (Report No 10). Canberra, AusInfo, 1999

Robins LN, Helzer JE, Croughan J, et al: National Institute of Mental Health Diagnostic Interview Schedule: its history, characteristics and validity. Arch Gen Psychiatry 38:381–389, 1981

Robins LN, Cottler LB, Compton WM, et al: The National Institute of Mental Health Diagnostic Interview Schedule (DIS),Version 4.0. St. Louis, MO, Washington University School of Medicine, Department of Psychiatry, 1997

Rose IN: Indian nations and Internet gambling. Casino City Times, October 22, 2000. Available at: http://rose.casinocitytimes.com/articles/969.html. Accessed November 28, 2003.

Shaffer HJ, Hall MN: Estimating the Prevalence of Disordered Gambling Behavior in the United States and Canada: A Meta-analysis. Boston, MA, President and Fellows of Harvard College, 1997

Shaffer HJ, Freed CR, Healea D: Gambling disorders among homeless persons with substance use disorders seeking treatment at a community center. Psychiatr Serv 53:1112–1117, 2002

Sproston K, Erens B, Orford J: The future of gambling in Britain (letter). BMJ 321:1291, 2000

Stinchfield R, Nadav C, Winters K, et al: Prevalence of gambling among Minnesota public school students in 1992 and 1995. J Gambl Stud 13:25–48, 1997

Taylor H: Internet Penetration at 66% of Adults (137 Million) Nationwide: 55% of Adults Now Online From Home and 30% Online at Work (Harris Poll #18, April 17, 2002). Rochester, NY, Harris Interactive, 2002. Available at: http://www.harrisinteractive.com/harris_poll/index.asp?PID=295. Accessed November 28, 2003.

Turner N: Internet gambling. Electronic Journal of Gambling Issues (6), 2002. Available at: http://www.camh.net/egambling/issue6/first_person/. Accessed November 29, 2003.

Volberg RA: The prevalence and demographics of pathological gamblers: implications for public health. Am J Public Health 84:237–241, 1994

Volberg RA: Gambling and Problem Gambling in Oregon: Report to the Oregon Gambling Addiction Treatment Foundation. Northampton, MA, Gemini Research, 1997

Volberg RA, Abbott MW: Gambling and problem gambling among indigenous people. Subst Use Misuse 32:1525–1538, 1997

Volberg RA, Abbott MW, Rönnberg S, et al: Prevalence and risks of pathological gambling in Sweden. Acta Psychiatr Scand 104:250–256, 2001

Wardman D, el-Guebaly N, Hodgins D: Problem and pathological gambling in North American Aboriginal populations: a review of the empirical literature. J Gambl Stud 17:81–100, 2001

Welte JB, Barnes GM, Wieczorek WF, et al: Gambling participation in the US—results from a national survey. J Gambl Stud 18:313–337, 2002

Westphal JR, Rush J: Pathological gambling in Louisiana: an epidemiological perspective. J La State Med Soc 148:353–358, 1996

Wharry S: You bet your life: e-gambling threat worries addiction experts (letter). CMAJ 165:325, 2001

Womack S, Compton W, Cottler LB: Internet/Computer Assessment Module–Self Administered (ICAM-SA). St. Louis, MO, Washington University School of Medicine, 2001

Womack SB, Cottler LB, Grucza RA, et al: Personality characteristics of Internet gamblers—preliminary results from the St. Louis Area Personality, Health and Lifestyle Survey 2001. Poster presentation at the Institute for Research on Pathological Gambling and Related Disorders Conference, Las Vegas, NV, December 8, 2002

Zane NWS, Huh-Kim J: Addictive behaviors, in Handbook of Asian American Psychology. Edited by Lee LC, Zane NWS. South Oaks, CA, Sage, 1998, pp 527–554

Zitzow D: Comparative study of problematic gambling behaviors between American Indian and non-Indian adolescents within and near a Northern Plains reservation. Am Indian Alsk Native Ment Health Res 7:14–26, 1996

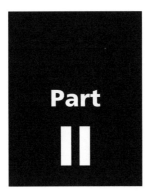

Part II

Clinical Characteristics

Clinical Characteristics

Tami R. Argo, Pharm.D.
Donald W. Black, M.D.

Mary, a 42-year-old accountant, had gambled recreationally for years. At age 38, for reasons she cannot explain, she became hooked on casino slot machines. Her interest in gambling gradually escalated, and within a year Mary was gambling during most business days. She also gambled most weekends, telling her husband she was at work. To acquire money for gambling, Mary created a fake company to which she transferred nearly $300,000 from her accounting firm. The embezzlement was eventually detected, and Mary was arrested. After her arrest and the associated public humiliation, Mary became severely depressed and attempted suicide by drug overdose. After a brief hospital stay, Mary entered counseling and was prescribed paroxetine. In a plea bargain, she agreed to perform 400 hours of community service.

Although in men, recreational gambling often begins during adolescence (Rosenthal 1992), women—like Mary in the case study above—tend to begin gambling later in life, often in their early 30s (Grant and Kim 2002; Tavares et al. 2001). Of course, not everyone who gambles recreationally develops pathological gambling. For many recreational gamblers, however, the development of pathological gambling may be precipitated by a major life stressor (Lesieur and Rosenthal 1991). Women tend to have a more rapid progression of pathological gambling, a phenomenon known as *telescoping.* In one study, the time interval from recreational gambling to problem gambling averaged 1 year in women and 4.6 years in men (Tavares et al. 2001). Gender differences are discussed more fully in Chapter 7, "Gender Differences."

g Course

v longitudinal studies have been reported, pathological gam-
ᴅ... med to be chronic, with a clinical course that is continuous,
unremitting, or episodic (Hollander et al. 2000a). Some researchers con-
tend that many pathological gamblers experience a big win early in their
gambling careers that directly results in their becoming addicted (Custer
and Milt 1985). Others cite the increased accessibility and exposure to
gambling-related activities as influencing the gradual progression from
recreational gambling to pathological gambling (Rosenthal 1992).

Pathological gambling has been characterized as a progressive, multi-
stage illness (Custer 1984). The first phase, called the *winning phase*, is
fostered by early successes and is more often found in men, perhaps reflecting a more competitive aspect of male gambling. Winning confers
feelings of status, power, and omnipotence. Features accompanying this
stage include high energy, focused concentration, improved ability with
numbers, and interest in gambling strategies. Many attribute their initial
winning to skill rather than to luck. Many gamblers are thought to derive
a substantial proportion of their self-esteem from gambling and rely on
gambling to help manage disappointments and negative mood states. The
gambler may begin to retreat from family and friends and may spend
more time and energy gambling. Fantasies of winning and thoughts of
great successes are typical.

Unexpected losses, often perceived as bad luck, lead to the second
phase, called the *losing phase*. This phase features *chasing*. The gambler
desperately tries to recover lost money by wagering more frequently and
in larger amounts. The gambler often lies to important persons (family
members, friends, and employers) to hide losses. Relationships generally
deteriorate and finances worsen. Eventually the gambler experiences a
crunch, in which legitimate sources of money have been exhausted. Family members may provide a financial bailout in exchange for promises to
stop gambling.

A spiraling pattern of losing and chasing losses leads to the third
phase, *desperation*. The gambler may engage in illegal activities such as
fraud, embezzlement, writing bad checks, or stealing to support his or
her gambling problem. Illegal behavior is rationalized, often with the in-
tent to repay funds after the big win that is thought to be imminent. Fantasies of escape and thoughts of suicide are reportedly common during
this phase (Lesieur and Rosenthal 1991).

Some gamblers experience a fourth phase of *giving up* or *hopelessness*.
The gambler may seek treatment, often at the insistence of their employer, spouse, or family members. Depression; thoughts of suicide; and

stress-related symptoms such as hypertension, palpitations, insomnia, and gastrointestinal distress may be reported (Rosenthal 1992).

Phenomenology

Grant and Kim (2001) described the clinical characteristics of a sample of 131 treatment-seeking pathological gamblers. The mean age was 31 years, and the sample included 60% women. The mean length of time from initial gambling to onset of pathological gambling was 6 years, with a range from 0 to 33 years. Nearly 50% progressed to pathological gambling within 1 year of beginning gambling; later onset of pathological gambling and the acknowledgment of gambling urges triggered by advertisements correlated with rapid progression. Subjects gambled about 16 hours per week and had lost nearly 45% of their income to gambling during the previous year. Their mean score on the South Oaks Gambling Screen (Lesieur and Blume 1987) was 14 (a score of 5 or higher indicates probable pathological gambling). All but one subject reported unsuccessful attempts to quit gambling, and 87% reported chasing. More than 80% reported gambling to escape dysphoria. Gamblers frequently reported lying to family and friends (44%), borrowing money to pay bills or buy food (30%), and reaching maximum credit limits (64%).

Illegal Behavior

Although complicated, an association between crime and pathological gambling is well established (Rosenthal and Lorenz 1992). The prevalence of criminal activity among pathological gamblers has been estimated to be between 20% and 80% (Blaszczynski et al. 1989; Brown 1987). In a sample of 109 treatment-seeking problem gamblers, 55% reported having committed gambling-related offenses, and 21% reported having been charged with a crime (Blaszczynski et al. 1989). The authors found a fourfold increase in illegal gambling-related behaviors (e.g., offenses designed to obtain money for gambling purposes). The estimated mean amount per gambling-related illegal offense was $4,091 (in Australian dollars; approximately $3,000 USD). Illegal behaviors reported include writing bad checks and engaging in embezzlement, larceny, tax fraud, or prostitution (in women) (Rosenthal 1992).

Despite the existence of a relationship between criminality and gambling, a causal nature of the relationship is still unclear. In the progression of pathological gambling, some gamblers (including Mary in the vignette presented above) resort to illegal acts to finance gambling or to pay outstanding debts. The addictive nature of pathological gambling may represent an important criminogenic factor (Meyer and Stadler 1999). Other work suggests that the need to maintain gambling is the primary motivation for criminal behavior (Lesieur 1979). As the gambler chases losses and exhausts legitimate sources of money, he or she often resorts to criminal behavior. As losses increase, the pressure to offend increases (Blaszczynski et al. 1989). In fact, gambling-related offenses may be associated with severity of pathological gambling, as demonstrated by involvement with multiple forms of gambling, owing debts to acquaintances, acknowledging gambling-related suicidality, reporting excessive substance use, and having received mental health treatment (Potenza et al. 2000).

Although an association exists between criminality and pathological gambling, personality features may be a common cause for both pathological gambling and criminality and thereby promote their co-occurrence. Antisocial personality disorder (ASPD) is more frequently found in pathological gamblers than in the general population (Cunningham-Williams et al. 1998). Problem gamblers reporting gambling-related arrest or incarceration were more likely to have features consistent with ASPD (Potenza et al. 2000). High rates of pathological gambling have been reported in prison settings. In a study of prison inmates in Nevada, 26% were considered to be probable pathological gamblers (Templer et al. 1993).

Emotional Consequences

Pathological gambling can adversely influence multiple life domains: social, financial, professional, and personal (National Opinion Research Center 1999). Persons may begin gambling as an enjoyable pastime or as a means of socialization. As gambling progresses, pathological gamblers may isolate themselves. Many experience a loss of control or feelings of guilt or shame related to gambling. A study of 131 pathological gamblers reported that more than 15% reported gambling-related marital problems (Grant and Kim 2001). Pathological gambling often erodes the trust of family members, particularly that of the spouse, leading to diminished intimacy (Moody 1990).

Pathological gambling often leads to work-related problems. Gambling urges may be frequent and difficult to control, resulting in absenteeism, poor performance, and job loss (National Opinion Research Center 1999). The loss of financial support associated with job loss can lead to desperate attempts to obtain funds, including exhausting one's own finances while chasing. Bankruptcy filings are relatively common (Potenza et al. 2000). In one study, 44% of pathological gamblers reported no savings or retirement funds, and 22% described losing their homes or automobiles or pawning valuables to cover gambling losses (Grant and Kim 2001).

Pathological gambling can lead to attempted or completed suicide. Attempted suicide has been reported in 17%–24% of Gamblers Anonymous members and individuals in treatment for pathological gambling (Potenza et al. 2000). A case series analyzing 44 completed gambling-related suicides in Australia showed that the majority of the victims were men, had a mean age of 40 years, and were either unemployed or from lower socioeconomic backgrounds. Nearly one-third had made at least one prior attempt, and 25% had sought some form of mental health treatment for problem gambling (Blaszczynski and Farrell 1998). Variables associated with completed suicide included depression, large financial debts, and relationship difficulties.

Psychiatric Comorbidity and Personality

Few investigators have studied rates of other psychiatric disorders in persons with pathological gambling, although pathological gamblers are reported to exhibit high rates of mood, anxiety, and substance use disorders (Table 3–1). For example, 76% of an inpatient sample admitted for pathological gambling met criteria for a current major depressive disorder (McCormick et al. 1984). In 25 problem gamblers recruited from a Gamblers Anonymous chapter, 72% reported experiencing major depression (Linden et al. 1986). Increased rates of bipolar disorder (lifetime prevalence of 24%) and hypomania (prevalence of 38%) have also been reported in persons with pathological gambling (Linden et al.1986; McCormick et al. 1984). Overall, 13%–78% of persons with pathological gambling are estimated to experience a mood disorder. Persons with pathological gambling also report high rates of lifetime anxiety disorders (Table 3–1). One study reported that nearly 20% of pathological gamblers met criteria for lifetime attention-deficit/hyperactivity disorder (Specker et al. 1995).

Rates of other impulse control disorders (ICDs) appear higher in persons with pathological gambling than in the general population. Investigators have reported rates ranging from 18% to 43% for one or more ICD (Black and Moyer 1998; Grant and Kim 2001; Specker et al. 1995). Compulsive shopping appears to be the most frequent comorbid ICD in persons with pathological gambling, perhaps because both compulsive shopping and pathological gambling have shared characteristics of focused attention, monetary gratification, and monetary exchange (Specker et al. 1995). Subjects with one ICD appear more likely to have a second, suggesting considerable overlap among the ICDs (Black et al. 1997; McElroy et al. 1991, 1994; Schlosser et al. 1994).

Table 3–1.   Comorbid Axis I psychiatric disorders in persons with pathological gambling

Study	Sample size	Assessment method	Mood disorders	Psychotic disorders	ADHD
McCormick et al. 1984	50	RDC	76%	N/A	N/A
Linden et al. 1986	25	SCID	72%	N/A	N/A
Bland et al. 1993	30	DIS	33%	0%	N/A
Specker et al. 1995	40	Operationalized diagnostic interview for ADHD; MIDI	N/A	N/A	20%
Specker et al. 1996	40	SCID	78%	3%	N/A
Black and Moyer 1998	30	DIS	60%	3%	40% (childhood conduct disorder)
Cunningham-Williams et al. 1998	161	DIS	MDD (9%); dysthymia (4%)	4%	N/A
Hollander et al. 1998	10	N/A	30% Bipolar disorder I and II*	*	20%
Hollander et al. 2000b	10	N/A	50%	N/A	N/A
Grant and Kim 2001	131	SCID-IV	34%	N/A	N/A
Zimmerman et al. 2002	15	SCID-IV; DID; BDI	53% Mania*	*	N/A

*Excluded condition.
Note. ADHD=attention-deficit/hyperactivity disorder; BDI=Beck Depression Inventory; DID=Diagnostic Inventory for Depression; DIS=Diagnostic Interview Schedule, Version III; GAD=generalized anxiety disorder; MDD=major depressive disorder; MIDI=Minnesota Impulsive Disorders Interview; N/A=not available; OCD=obsessive-compulsive disorder; RDC=Research Diagnostic Criteria; SCID=Structured Clinical Interview for DSM-III; SCID-IV=Structured Clinical Interview for DSM-IV.

OCD	Substance use disorders	Eating disorders	Impulse control disorders	Anxiety disorders	No disorder
N/A	36%	N/A	N/A	N/A	N/A
20%	48%	N/A	N/A	28%	N/A
17%	63%	N/A	N/A	27%	N/A
N/A	N/A	N/A	35%	N/A	N/A
3%	60%	N/A	N/A	38%	8%
10%	63%	7%	43%	40%	N/A
1%	Alcohol (45%); illicit drugs (40%)	N/A	N/A	Panic disorder (23%); GAD (8%); phobias (15%)	N/A
10%	Current*	N/A	N/A	N/A	50%
10%	10%	N/A	N/A	20%	N/A
0%	35%	N/A	18%	9%	N/A
N/A	Current*	N/A	N/A	20%	N/A

Table 3–2. Comorbid personality disorders in persons with pathological gambling

Study	Sample size	Assessment method	Any PD	Paranoid	Schizoid	Schizotypal
Blaszczynski et al. 1989	109	DSM-III criteria	N/A	N/A	N/A	N/A
Lesieur and Blume 1990	7	N/A	71%	N/A	N/A	28%
Bellaire and Caspari 1992	51	N/A	N/A	N/A	N/A	N/A
Bland et al. 1993	30	DIS	N/A	N/A	N/A	N/A
Specker et al. 1996	40	SCID-P	25%	3%	3%	0%
Black and Moyer 1998	30	PDQ-R	87%	26%	33%	30%
Blaszczynski and Steel 1998	82	PDQ-R	93%	40%	21%	38%

Note. ASPD=antisocial personality disorder; BPD=borderline personality disorder; DIS=Diagnostic Interview Schedule, Version III; N/A=not available; NOS=not otherwise specified; OCPD=obsessive-compulsive personality disorder; PD=personality disorder; PDQ-R=Personality Disorders Questionnaire–Revised; SCID-P=Structured Clinical Interview for DSM-III Personality Disorders.

Lifetime alcohol or drug dependence has been consistently reported in persons with pathological gambling. Twenty-eight percent of persons with pathological gambling had current alcohol dependence, compared with a rate of 1% for nonpathological gamblers (Welte et al. 2001). In its study, the National Opinion Research Center (1999) found that among persons with pathological gambling, the rate of alcohol or other drug abuse was nearly seven times higher than that among nongamblers or recreational gamblers. Up to 30%–50% of treatment-seeking pathological gamblers have histories of substance abuse (Lesieur et al. 1986).

Rates of pathological gambling are higher than expected among inpatients being treated for substance abuse. Among 462 patients enrolled in methadone maintenance programs, 21% were probable pathological gamblers (Spunt et al. 1998). The Epidemiologic Catchment Area study indicated that problem gambling occurred within 2 years of the onset of alcoholism in 65% of gambling cases (Cunningham-Williams et al. 1998). The available studies support a significant association between substance use and pathological gambling. There may be subgroups (e.g., based on gender or psychiatric status) in which the development of co-

BPD	Histrionic	Narcissistic	Avoidant	OCPD	ASPD	Dependent	Unspecified
14%	N/A	N/A	N/A	N/A	N/A	N/A	14%
N/A	N/A	N/A	N/A	N/A	N/A	N/A	49%
N/A	N/A	N/A	N/A	N/A	15%	N/A	N/A
N/A	N/A	N/A	N/A	N/A	40%	N/A	N/A
3%	0%	5%	13%	5%	0%	5%	3%
23%	7%	20%	50%	59%	17%	7%	N/A
70%	66%	57%	37%	32%	29%	49%	N/A

occurrence is more or less likely; however, the variables marking such subgroups have yet to be firmly established.

Personality Disorders

Personality disorders in pathological gambling have been relatively unexplored, despite the fact that early psychoanalysts described pathological gambling as a neurosis and individuals with pathological gambling as being guilt-ridden, narcissistic, or masochistic. Both Kraepelin (1915) and Bleuler (1924) described "gambling mania" as an example of an impulsive neurosis. Freud (1928/1961) interpreted compulsive gambling as a form of self-castigation, and Bergler (1957) interpreted excessive gambling as a form of "psychic masochism." He believed that a person engaged in gambling unconsciously punished himself through the guilt and anxiety that followed losing.

Although these views shaped early assessments of pathological gambling, later systematic studies have found that personality disorders are relatively common in persons with pathological gambling (Table 3–2). Based on limited information available, a small but significant subset of pathological gamblers have ASPD. Rates of ASPD range from 15% to 40%, compared with rates of 3% of males and 1% of females in the general population (American Psychiatric Association 1994; Black and

Moyer 1998; Bland et al. 1993; Blaszczynski and Steel 1998; Blaszczynski et al. 1989). Although other types of personality disorders may be present in persons with pathological gambling, their rates are generally no higher than those in the general population.

Dimensional Personality Traits and Characteristics

Personality traits and characteristics are present along a spectrum and may be better measured dimensionally, with diagnosable personality disorder at one extreme. Roy et al. (1989) found that a group of pathological gamblers had higher scores than control subjects on the neuroticism, psychoticism, and lie scales of the Eysenck Personality Questionnaire (Eysenck and Eysenck 1980) and that they achieved higher scores on the hostility scale of the Foulds questionnaire (Foulds 1965). The investigators concluded that persons with pathological gambling can be moody, nervous, sensitive, attention seeking, and hostile. Elevations on the psychopathic deviation scale of the Minnesota Multiphasic Personality Inventory (MMPI) have been reported, supporting clinical impressions relating pathological gambling and ASPD (Graham and Lowenfeld 1986; Moravec and Munley 1983; Taber et al. 1987; Templer et al. 1993). Elevations have also been reported on the depression, paranoia, psychasthenia, and schizophrenia scales of the MMPI (Graham and Lowenfeld 1986; Templer et al. 1993). Researchers have reported increased rates of alexithymia, attentional impairment, impulsiveness, risk taking, obsessionality, sensation seeking, lack of behavioral restraint, diminished ability to resist craving, poor coping, negative affect, and novelty seeking in persons with pathological gambling compared with normative samples (Blaszczynski 1999; Carlton and Manowitz 1992; Castellani and Rugle 1995; Castellani et al. 1996; Coventry and Brown 1993; Kim and Grant 2001; Kusyszyn and Rutter 1985; Lumley and Roby 1995; McCormick 1993; Powell et al. 1999). These wide-ranging traits appear to describe individuals who seek excitement and new experiences, easily submit to their desires, and exercise little restraint over their impulses.

Subtypes

Recognizing the heterogeneity of pathological gambling, some researchers have attempted to identify subtypes of pathological gambling. Moran (1970) identified five subtypes based on work with 50 pathological gamblers (Table 3–3). Although Moran's typology is clinically useful, it has not been empirically validated, and the subtypes are not discrete.

Table 3–3. Five subtypes of pathological gamblers

Type	Prevalence	Description
Neurotic gambling	34%	Gambling is motivated in response to an emotional problem, such as marital conflict, and subsides when the conflict is resolved.
Psychopathic gambling	24%	Gambling appears as an antisocial behavioral pattern.
Impulsive gambling	18%	Gambling is accompanied by a loss of control.
Subcultural gambling	14%	The person gambles to fit in with peers but later has difficulty controlling gambling.
Symptomatic gambling	10%	Gambling is associated with some other mental illness, such as depression, and is considered a secondary phenomenon.

Source. Moran 1970.

Steel and Blaszczynski (1996) used principal-components analysis to investigate the factorial structure of pathological gambling. They identified four primary factors described in Table 3–4. The investigators concluded that pathological gamblers exhibiting features of impulsivity and ASPD are at greatest risk for experiencing adverse personal and emotional consequences.

Table 3–4. Four primary factors of pathological gambling

Factor	Associated trait(s)
Psychological distress	Female gender Suicidality Family psychiatric history
Sensation seeking	History of alcohol abuse
Crime and liveliness	Criminal activity
Impulsivity and antisocial behavioral patterns[a]	Early onset of gambling Poor job history Separation or divorce due to gambling Impulsive gambling-related illegal acts

[a]Described as the most clinically useful.
Source. Steel and Blaszczynski 1996.

Conclusion

Despite relatively low prevalence estimates, pathological gambling has the potential to cause significant dysfunction for the gambler and those in his or her relationships, including spouses, family members, friends, and coworkers. Pathological gamblers generally exhibit high levels of novelty seeking and impulsiveness. Comorbid psychiatric disorders are common—particularly mood, anxiety, and substance use disorders; other ICDs; and ASPD. Future investigations into the course of pathological gambling and its relationship to patterns of comorbid disorders have the potential to lead to improved treatment strategies (see Chapter 13, "Pharmacological Treatments").

References

American Psychiatric Association: Diagnostic and Statistical Manual of Mental Disorders, 4th Edition. Washington, DC, American Psychiatric Association, 1994

Bellaire W, Caspari D: Diagnosis and therapy of male gamblers in a university psychiatric hospital. J Gambl Stud 8:143–150, 1992

Bergler E: The Psychiatry of Gambling. New York, Hill & Wang, 1957

Black DW, Moyer T: Clinical features and psychiatric comorbidity of subjects with pathological gambling behavior. Psychiatr Serv 49:1434–1439, 1998

Black DW, Kehrberg LLD, Flumerfelt DL, et al: Characteristics of 36 subjects reporting compulsive sexual behavior. Am J Psychiatry 154:243–249, 1997

Bland RC, Newman SC, Orn H, et al: Epidemiology of pathological gambling in Edmonton. Can J Psychiatry 38:108–112, 1993

Blaszczynski A: Pathological gambling and obsessive-compulsive spectrum disorders. Psychol Rep 84:107–113, 1999

Blaszczynski A, Farrell E: A case series of 44 completed gambling-related suicides. J Gambl Stud 14:93–109, 1998

Blaszczynski A, Steel Z: Personality disorders among pathological gamblers. J Gambl Stud 14:51–71, 1998

Blaszczynski A, McConaghy N, Frankova A: Crime, antisocial personality, and pathological gambling. Journal of Gambling Behavior 5:137–152, 1989

Bleuler E: Textbook of Psychiatry. New York, Macmillan, 1924

Brown RIF: Pathological gambling and associated patterns of crime: comparisons with alcohol and other drug addictions. Journal of Gambling Behavior 3:98–114, 1987

Carlton PL, Manowitz P: Behavioral restraint and symptoms of attention deficit disorder in alcoholics and pathological gamblers. Neuropsychobiology 25:44–48, 1992

Castellani B, Rugle L: A comparison of pathological gamblers to alcoholics and cocaine misusers on impulsivity, sensation seeking, and craving. Int J Addict 30:275–289, 1995

Castellani B, Wootton E, Rugle L, et al: Homelessness, negative affect, and coping among veterans with gambling problems who misused substances. Psychiatr Serv 47:298–299, 1996

Coventry KR, Brown RIF: Sensation seeking, gambling and gambling addictions. Addiction 88:541–554, 1993

Cunningham-Williams RM, Cottler LB, Compton WM III, et al: Taking chances: problem gamblers and mental health disorders—results from the St. Louis Epidemiologic Catchment Area Study. Am J Public Health 88:1093–1096, 1998

Custer RL: Profile of the pathological gambler. J Clin Psychiatry 45:35–38, 1984

Custer RL, Milt H: When Luck Runs Out. New York, Facts on File, 1985

Eysenck H, Eysenck S: Manual of the Eysenck Personality Questionnaire. London, Hodder & Stroughton, 1980

Foulds G: Personality and Personal Illness. London, Tavistock, 1965

Freud S: Dostoevsky and parricide (1928), in The Standard Edition of the Complete Psychological Works of Sigmund Freud, Vol 21. Translated and edited by Strachey J. London, Hogarth Press, 1961, pp 175–196

Graham JR, Lowenfeld BH: Personality dimensions of the pathological gambler. Journal of Gambling Behavior 2:58–66, 1986

Grant JE, Kim SW: Demographic and clinical features of 131 adult pathological gamblers. J Clin Psychiatry 62:957–962, 2001

Grant JE, Kim SW: Gender differences in pathological gamblers seeking medication treatment. Compr Psychiatry 43:56–62, 2002

Hollander E, DeCaria CM, Mari E, et al: Short-term single-blind fluvoxamine treatment of pathological gambling. Am J Psychiatry 155:1781–1783, 1998

Hollander E, Buchalter AJ, DeCaria C: Pathological gambling. Psychiatr Clin North Am 23:629–642, 2000a

Hollander E, DeCaria CM, Finkell JN, et al: A randomized double-blind fluvoxamine/placebo crossover trial in pathologic gambling. Biol Psychiatry 47:813–817, 2000b

Kim SW, Grant JE: Personality dimensions in pathological gambling disorder and obsessive-compulsive disorder. Psychiatry Res 104:205–212, 2001

Kraepelin E: Psychiatrie, 8th Edition. Leipzig, Verlag von Johann Ambrosius Barth, 1915

Kusyszyn I, Rutter R: Personality characteristics of male heavy gamblers, light gamblers, nongamblers, and lottery players. Journal of Gambling Behavior 1:59–63, 1985

Lesieur HR: The compulsive gambler's spiral of options and involvement. Psychiatry 42:79–87, 1979

Lesieur HR, Blume SE: The South Oaks Gambling Screen (SOGS): a new instrument for identification of pathological gamblers. Am J Psychiatry 144:1184–1188, 1987

Lesieur HR, Blume SB: Characteristics of pathological gamblers identified among patients on a psychiatric admissions service. Hosp Community Psychiatry 41:1009–1012, 1990

Lesieur HR, Rosenthal RJ: Pathological gambling: a review of the literature. J Gambl Stud 7:5–39, 1991

Lesieur HR, Blume SB, Zoppa RM: Alcoholism, drug abuse, and gambling. Alcohol Clin Exp Res 10:33–38, 1986

Linden RD, Pope HG Jr, Jonas JM: Pathological gambling and major affective disorder: preliminary findings. J Clin Psychiatry 47:201–203, 1986

Lumley MA, Roby KT: Alexithymia and pathological gambling. Psychother Psychosom 63:201–206, 1995

McCormick RA: Disinhibition and negative affectivity in substance abusers with and without a gambling problem. Addict Behav 18:331–336, 1993

McCormick RA, Russo AM, Ramirez LF, et al: Affective disorders among pathological gamblers seeking treatment. Am J Psychiatry 141:215–218, 1984

McElroy SL, Pope HG Jr, Hudson JL, et al: Kleptomania: a report of 20 cases. Am J Psychiatry 148:652–657, 1991

McElroy SL, Keck PE Jr, Pope HG Jr, et al: Compulsive buying: a report of 20 cases. J Clin Psychiatry 55:242–248, 1994

Meyer G, Stadler MA: Criminal behavior associated with pathological gambling. J Gambl Stud 15:29–43, 1999

Moody G: Quit Compulsive Gambling: The Action Plan for Gamblers and Their Families. Wellingborough, UK, Thorsons, 1990

Moran E: Varieties of pathological gambling. Br J Psychiatry 116:593–597, 1970

Moravec JD, Munley PH: Psychological test findings on pathological gamblers in treatment. Int J Addict 18:1003–1009, 1983

National Opinion Research Center: Gambling Impact and Behavior Study: Report to the National Gambling Impact Study Commission. Chicago, IL, National Opinion Research Center at the University of Chicago, 1999. Available at: http://www.norc.uchicago.edu/new/gamb-fin.htm. Accessed December 13, 2003.

Potenza MN, Steinberg MA, McLaughlin SD, et al: Illegal behaviors in problem gambling: analysis of data from a gambling helpline. J Am Acad Psychiatry Law 28:389–403, 2000

Powell J, Hardoon K, Derevensky JL, et al: Gambling and risk-taking behavior among university students. Subst Use Misuse 34:1167–1184, 1999

Rosenthal RJ: Pathological gambling. Psychiatr Ann 22:72–78, 1992

Rosenthal RJ, Lorenz VC: The pathological gambler as criminal offender. Comments on evaluation and treatment. Psychiatr Clin North Am 15:647–660, 1992

Roy A, Custer R, Lorenz V, et al: Personality factors and pathological gambling. Acta Psychiatr Scand 80:37–39, 1989

Schlosser S, Black DW, Repertinger S, et al: Compulsive buying: demography, phenomenology, and comorbidity in 46 subjects. Gen Hosp Psychiatry 16:205–212, 1994

Specker SM, Carlson GA, Christenson GA, et al: Impulse control disorders and attention deficit disorder in pathological gamblers. Ann Clin Psychiatry 7:175–179, 1995

Specker SM, Carlson GA, Edmonson KM, et al: Psychopathology in pathological gamblers seeking treatment. J Gambl Stud 12:67–81, 1996

Spunt B, Dupont I, Lesieur H, et al: Pathological gambling and substance abuse: a review of the literature. Subst Use Misuse 33:2535–2560, 1998

Steel Z, Blaszczynski A: The factorial structure of pathological gambling. J Gambl Stud 12:3–20, 1996

Taber JI, McCormick RA, Russo AM, et al: Follow-up of pathological gamblers after treatment. Am J Psychiatry 144:757–761, 1987

Tavares H, Zilberman ML, Beites FJ, et al: Gender differences in gambling progression. J Gambl Stud 17:151–159, 2001

Templer DI, Kaiser G, Siscoe K: Correlates of pathological gambling propensity in prison inmates. Compr Psychiatry 34:347–351, 1993

Welte J, Barnes G, Wieczorek W, et al: Alcohol and gambling pathology among U.S. adults: prevalence, demographic patterns and comorbidity. J Stud Alcohol 62:706–712, 2001

Zimmerman M, Breen RB, Posternak MA: An open-label study of citalopram in the treatment of pathological gambling. J Clin Psychiatry 63:44–48, 2002

Categorization

Paula Moreyra, M.A.
Angela Ibáñez, M.D., Ph.D.
Jerónimo Saiz-Ruiz, M.D., Ph.D.
Carlos Blanco, M.D., Ph.D.

Pathological gambling is classified in DSM-IV-TR (American Psychiatric Association 2000) as an impulse control disorder not elsewhere classified. However, there is evidence that it also shares features of obsessive-compulsive, substance use, and mood disorders. Because the conceptualization of pathological gambling will likely influence research and treatment models, an understanding of data supporting each conceptualization is important.

Impulse Control Disorder

Characteristics of impulse control disorders (ICDs) that are recognizable in pathological gambling include a desire or temptation to perform some behavior (gambling) despite its detrimental consequences for the individual or others; a progressive emotional discomfort or tension before performing the act; pleasurable or gratifying feelings while performing the behavior (i.e., gambling is ego-syntonic); and, in some cases, negative feelings of guilt, remorse, or shame following the behavior (American Psychiatric Association 1994; World Health Organization 1992). Data supporting the categorization of pathological gambling as an ICD include elevated rates of comorbid ICDs among pathological gamblers (Black and Moyer 1998; Specker et al. 1995). Although the samples were relatively small, subjects reported high rates of comorbid compulsive sexual disorder, intermittent explosive disorder, and compulsive buying. A study of 96 pathological gamblers found similarly elevated rates of ICDs. Pathological gamblers with comorbid ICDs reported more intense urges to gamble compared with those without comorbid ICDs, and this finding suggests a common neurobiology for ICDs (Grant and Kim 2003).

Despite similarities among ICDs, pathological gambling has unique features. For example, in pathological gambling impulsivity is arguably limited to a single activity (gambling), and this differentiates pathological gambling from other disorders (such as bipolar disorder) in which the impulsivity may be more generalized. Among models that closely relate impulsivity with specific thoughts or activities are conceptualizations of pathological gambling as an obsessive-compulsive spectrum disorder or as a nonpharmacological addiction (Table 4–1).

Substance Use Disorder

One model proposed for pathological gambling is as an addiction without the drug. Pathological gambling and substance use disorders share many features: an intense desire to satisfy a need, loss of control over the substance use or behavior, periods of abstinence and tolerance, thoughts about the use of the substance or related activities, and continued engagement in the behavior despite significant social and occupational problems related to it (World Health Organization 1992).

A pathological gambler's desire to bet may be analogous to cravings experienced by substance abusers. A study of 854 substance abusers and pathological gamblers suggested that pathological gamblers had more difficulties resisting gambling urges than substance abusers had resisting drug cravings (Castellani and Rugle 1995). Approximately one-third of pathological gamblers experience irritability, psychomotor agitation, difficulties concentrating, and other somatic complaints following periods of gambling, features that share similarities with withdrawal symptoms (Dickerson 1989; Wray et al. 1981).

Pathological gamblers often increase the frequency of their bets or the amount of money they gamble to achieve the desired level of excitement. This behavior is suggestive of drug tolerance. Pathological gamblers may become preoccupied with gambling-related activities (Lesieur 1979) despite negative domestic, professional, financial, and social consequences of their gambling (Bland et al. 1993).

Table 4–1. Common features shared by pathological gambling and other disorders

	Impulse control disorders	Substance use disorders	Obsessive-compulsive spectrum disorders	Affective disorders
Phenomenology	Difficulty resisting impulses, desire to act despite negative consequences, alleviation of emotional discomfort when act is performed	Several DSM-IV-TR criteria, including continued behavior despite interference in life functioning, multiple unsuccessful attempts to diminish or stop behavior, and symptoms of tolerance and withdrawal	Some DSM-IV-TR criteria, such as repetitive thoughts and diminished ability to resist urges	Harmful yet pleasurable behavior, acting without forethought, and mood fluctuations
Comorbidity	Elevated rates of impulse control disorders among pathological gamblers	High rates of comorbidity of multiple substance use disorders, particularly alcohol abuse and dependence and nicotine dependence	Some suggestion of elevated rates of OCD among pathological gamblers, with large studies generally finding no increased comorbidity	Increased rates of comorbid depressive disorders and high rates of suicide attempts
Epidemiology	Insufficient information	Prevalence in males; elevated rates of ADHD	Insufficient information	Insufficient information
Genetics	Insufficient information	Association between polymorphisms of DRD2, MAOA, and SLC6A4	Insufficient information	Insufficient information

Table 4–1. Common features shared by pathological gambling and other disorders *(continued)*

	Impulse control disorders	Substance use disorders	Obsessive-compulsive spectrum disorders	Affective disorders
Neuropsychology	Deficits in higher-order attention capacities; high impulsivity	Deficits in higher-order attention capacities; high impulsivity	Insufficient information	Insufficient information
Treatment response	Positive response to naltrexone documented in kleptomania and compulsive buying	Positive responses to naltrexone, 12-step programs, and interventions with relapse prevention	Positive responses to SSRIs	Positive responses to lithium and carbamazepine

Note. ADHD=attention-deficit/hyperactivity disorder; OCD=obsessive-compulsive disorder; SSRI=selective serotonin reuptake inhibitor.

Further support for the categorization of pathological gambling as a nonpharmacological addiction is the high comorbidity between pathological gambling and substance use disorders, particularly alcohol abuse and dependence. Estimates of substance abuse among pathological gamblers range from 10% to 52%, and to 85% if nicotine is included (Daghestani et al. 1996; Haberman 1969; Lesieur and Heineman 1988; Lesieur et al. 1986; Linden et al. 1986; McCormick et al. 1984; Spunt et al. 1995; Volberg 1996). Conversely, substance abusers show high rates of pathological gambling, ranging from 9% to 33% (Daghestani et al. 1996; Haberman 1969; Lesieur et al. 1986; Spunt et al. 1995; Volberg 1996). This association may be due to common etiological mechanisms or the frequent presence and use of substances in gambling venues.

Preliminary molecular genetic findings suggest commonalities between pathological gambling and substance use disorders. Specifically, an association between polymorphisms of the dopamine D$_2$ receptor gene *(DRD2)*, the monoamine oxidase A gene *(MAOA)*, and the serotonin transporter gene *(SLC6A4)* have been similarly reported in pathological gamblers and substance abusers (Blum et al. 1995; Comings et al. 1996; Ibáñez et al. 2000; Perez de Castro et al. 1999). Although roles for dopaminergic and serotonergic pathways in substance abuse are widely accepted, data on a role for dopamine in pathological gambling are more limited (see Chapter 9, "Biological Basis for Pathological Gambling").

Neuropsychological testing supports a substance use model of pathological gambling. Pathological gamblers have deficits in higher-order attention capacities related to the maintenance of goal-directed programs, planning, sequencing, and sustaining inhibitory control over distracting stimuli (Rugle and Melamed 1993). These deficits are similar to those found in substance abusers (Rosselli and Ardila 1996).

The association of pathological gambling and substance use disorders may be mediated by other factors such as gender, comorbidity, or personality dimensions. Epidemiological studies indicate that approximately two-thirds of pathological gamblers are male. Similarly, substance abuse is more prevalent in males, indicating that the pattern of prevalence according to gender is similar in both disorders (Cunningham-Williams et al. 1998; Volberg 1994; Warner et al. 1995).

Data suggest that attention-deficit/hyperactivity disorder (ADHD) is associated with both pathological gambling and substance use disorders (Carlton and Manowitz 1988; Carlton et al. 1987; Specker et al. 1995). Individuals with ADHD appear to be at increased risk of developing a substance use disorder (Biederman et al. 1995; Mannuzza et al. 1993).

Pathological gamblers have elevated measures of impulsivity, and this impulsivity is related to gambling severity (Blaszczynski et al. 1997; Carlton and Manowitz 1994; Castellani and Rugle 1995; Steel and Blaszczynski 1998). Similarly, a correlation has been found between levels of impulsivity and substance abuse or its risk (Allen et al. 1998). In individuals with a substance use disorder and pathological gambling, impulsivity may underlie both behaviors. Studies suggest that substance abusers with gambling problems are more impulsive (as measured by more rapid temporal discounting of rewards) than are those without gambling problems (Petry and Casarella 1999), and pathological gamblers with and without substance use disorders discount rewards at high rates (Petry 2001).

Similarities between pathological gambling and substance abuse are suggested by treatment studies. Naltrexone, a treatment for opiate and alcohol dependence approved by the U.S. Food and Drug Administration, has shown preliminary efficacy in the treatment of pathological gambling (see Chapter 13, "Pharmacological Treatments"). Mixed findings have been observed for the use of selective serotonin reuptake inhibitors (SSRIs) in the treatment of pathological gambling (see Chapter 13) and substance use disorders (Angelone et al. 1998; Cornelius et al. 1997; Kabel and Petty 1996; Kranzler et al. 1995).

Data suggest that pathological gamblers may respond similarly to participation in 12-step programs (e.g., Gamblers Anonymous) as do individuals with substance use disorders who participate in self-help programs (e.g., Alcoholics Anonymous or Narcotics Anonymous) (Potenza et al. 2001). Cognitive-behavioral therapies analogous to those used for relapse prevention in substance use disorders have demonstrated preliminary efficacy in controlled treatment trials (see Chapter 12, "Cognitive and Behavioral Treatments"). Because relapse after treatment is common in substance abuse and pathological gambling, cognitive-behavioral approaches often rely on models of relapse prevention that advocate the recognition and avoidance of cues leading to the addictive behavior and the development of alternative coping strategies to achieve and maintain abstinence (Marlatt and Gordon 1985).

In summary, data from phenomenology and epidemiology strongly suggest a link between pathological gambling and substance abuse (see Table 4–1). However, these data often do not provide information regarding the nature of that relationship. Future studies, particularly those in the areas of genetics, neuropsychology, and treatment response, will likely generate an improved understanding of the precise mechanisms linking pathological gambling and substance use disorders.

Obsessive-Compulsive Spectrum Disorder

An alternative conceptualization for pathological gambling is as an obsessive-compulsive spectrum disorder (see Table 4–1). It has been suggested that obsessive-compulsive spectrum disorders may share phenomenological, genetic, and other biological features (Stein 2000) with pathological gambling. Patients with obsessive-compulsive spectrum disorders experience unpleasant feelings and a physiological activation that results in an intense desire to perform a specific behavior to relieve the unpleasant feelings (Cartwright et al. 1998; Hantouche and Merckaert 1991; Hollander et al. 1996). Repetitive gambling and the gambling-related thoughts of pathological gambling are consistent with characteristics found in other obsessive-compulsive spectrum disorders. Data suggest that a diminished ability to resist gambling thoughts leads to excessive gambling, especially in advanced phases of pathological gambling (Lesieur 1979).

Other data do not support the categorization of pathological gambling as an obsessive-compulsive spectrum disorder. Although gambling and the related thoughts are often ego-syntonic for pathological gamblers, obsessions and compulsions are generally ego-dystonic in obsessive-compulsive disorder (OCD). Patients with OCD frequently experience excessive doubt, a feature that is not characteristic of pathological gamblers (American Psychiatric Association 2000; Hollander et al. 1996; Lesieur and Custer 1984; Rasmussen and Eisen 1992). The compulsions of OCD are characterized by an increased sense of harm avoidance, risk aversion, and anticipatory anxiety (Rasmussen and Eisen 1992). Pathological gamblers do not display these characteristics (Kim and Grant 2001; Lesieur and Custer 1984).

Epidemiological studies examining the comorbidity of OCD and pathological gambling have had mixed results, with some studies observing an association (Bland et al. 1993) and others not (Cunningham-Williams et al. 1998). In a small sample of pathological gamblers, 20% met diagnostic criteria for OCD, but more than half of those met additional criteria for alcohol abuse or bipolar disorder, complicating the interpretation of the results (Linden et al. 1986). A recent study found no subjects with current or past pathological gambling in a group of 80 patients with OCD and only one subject with pathological gambling in a group of 343 first-degree relatives of patients with OCD (Bienvenu et al. 2000). Similarly, a study of more than 700 individuals with OCD did not find elevated rates of pathological gambling (Hollander et al. 1997).

Harm avoidance, elevated in OCD, contrasts with the risk-seeking behavior characteristic of pathological gambling. Obsessive-compulsive behaviors and impulsivity, however, are not mutually exclusive (Stein 2000; Stein and Hollander 1993). Examination of impulsivity in patients with OCD has been inconclusive. One study found no significant difference in impulsivity scores between a group of patients with OCD and a group of control subjects (Stein et al. 1994). In contrast, a study comparing patients with OCD and a history of poor impulse control with non-impulsive OCD patients found that the impulsive OCD patients scored significantly higher on impulsivity (Hoehn-Saric and Barksdale 1983), suggesting that a subgroup of patients with OCD may have high impulsivity.

Using the Padua Inventory, one study found that pathological gamblers scored significantly higher than social gamblers on obsessive-compulsive measures. The "obsessional" quality of the pathological gamblers, however, was due to elevated scores on two factors: "impaired control over mental activities" and "urges and worries of losing control over motor behaviors" (Blaszczynski 1999). Because loss of control over gambling defines pathological gambling, it is questionable whether these two factors reflect an obsessional quality of pathological gamblers or an adequate assessment of reality.

The Tridimensional Personality Questionnaire, which assesses three personality dimensions (novelty seeking, reward dependence, and harm avoidance), was administered to a group of subjects with either pathological gambling or OCD (Kim and Grant 2001). Subjects with pathological gambling expressed greater novelty seeking, impulsiveness, and extravagance and less anticipatory worry, fear of uncertainty, and harm avoidance than the subjects with OCD.

Regarding treatments, SSRIs are effective for OCD (Pigott and Seay 1999), and preliminary evidence suggests their efficacy in treating pathological gambling. Cognitive-behavioral therapy is an established treatment for OCD and is an emerging treatment for pathological gambling (see Chapter 12, "Cognitive and Behavioral Treatments"). There are some differences in the types of cognitive-behavioral therapy used for the disorders. The cognitive-behavioral therapy used in OCD is based on a model of exposure and prevention of response (Foa et al. 1998). Existing cognitive-behavioral treatments for pathological gambling either emphasize the cognitive component (Sylvain et al. 1997) or are modeled on relapse-prevention strategies used in the treatment of substance use disorders (Petry and Roll 2001). As such, cognitive-behavioral therapy protocols in the treatment of pathological gambling more closely resemble those used for substance use disorders than those used for OCD treatment.

Affective Disorder

An alternative conceptualization for pathological gambling is as an affective spectrum disorder (see Table 4–1). Support for this categorization is derived from high rates of lifetime depression in persons with pathological gambling, ranging up to 76% (Cusack et al. 1993; Linden et al. 1986; McCormick et al. 1984; Sullivan et al. 1994). Elevated ratings of depression have been exhibited by pathological gamblers (Blaszczynski and McConaghy 1988; McCormick et al. 1987; Saiz-Ruiz et al. 1992), although many early studies lacked standard assessment instruments. A recent study using structured interviews suggested a relatively low occurrence of major depressive disorder in pathological gambling but a high occurrence of adjustment disorders with depressed mood (Ibáñez et al. 2001). An association between depression and pathological gambling does not establish causality or necessarily suggest a common etiology. Mood symptoms associated with pathological gambling could constitute a secondary reaction to negative consequences of gambling (Moreno et al. 1995; Saiz-Ruiz and Lopez-Ibor 1993; Saiz-Ruiz et al. 1992; Sullivan et al. 1994; Thorson et al. 1994).

Elevated rates of suicide attempts among persons with pathological gambling support its conceptualization as an affective spectrum disorder (McCormick et al. 1984; Saiz-Ruiz and Lopez-Ibor 1993). A study of treatment-seeking pathological gamblers reported that 49% had a history of suicidal ideation or suicide attempts (Petry and Kiluk 2002). Another study found that 90% of 167 pathological gamblers had experienced suicidal ideation (Sullivan et al. 1994). Whether these rates of suicidal ideation generalize to the larger population of non-treatment-seeking pathological gamblers is unknown. High rates of suicidality in pathological gambling do not necessarily constitute a direct link with depression, because other mental health disorders that are distinct from depression (e.g., schizophrenia) have high rates of suicidality. High levels of impulsiveness, often reported in association with pathological gambling, may lead to suicidality independent of depression. As such, there exists a need for further research to clarify the relationship between suicidality, impulsiveness, mood, and pathological gambling.

ICDs, such as pathological gambling, may represent bipolar spectrum disorders (McElroy et al. 1996). These disorders involve potentially harmful but pleasurable behaviors and acting without forethought. Similar to patients with bipolar disorder, pathological gamblers may experience mood fluctuations, although those fluctuations appear more marked in the case of bipolar disorders than in pathological gambling. These disorders generally have their onset in early adulthood and have an episodic course.

Based on the conceptualization of pathological gambling as an affective spectrum disorder, treatment modalities known to be successful for these disorders, including lithium and carbamazepine, have been tried successfully in individual cases (Haller and Hinterhuber 1994; Moskowitz 1980). Using single-blind designs, Pallanti and coworkers (2002) found lithium and valproate to be efficacious in non-bipolar pathological gamblers. Whether improvement of gambling behavior was due to the mood-stabilizing properties of these medications, their effect on impulsivity, or some other mechanism is not currently known.

Conclusion

Throughout the chapter, we have adopted the perspective that pathological gambling is a homogeneous entity with similar phenomenology, etiology, and treatment responsiveness. An alternative view is to consider pathological gambling as a heterogeneous disorder with subtypes that share certain characteristics. Future research should assess phenomenological aspects of gambling such as the choice of the gambling setting and activity, the motivations to gamble, and mood states during gambling. Studies of the natural history of pathological gambling, differential treatment responses, and underlying neurobiological differences could help define subgroups of pathological gamblers and guide prevention and treatment efforts.

References

Allen TJ, Moeller FG, Rhoades HM, et al: Impulsivity and history of drug dependence. Drug Alcohol Depend 50:137–145, 1998

American Psychiatric Association: Diagnostic and Statistical Manual of Mental Disorders, 4th Edition. Washington, DC, American Psychiatric Association, 1994

American Psychiatric Association: Diagnostic and Statistical Manual of Mental Disorders, 4th Edition, Text Revision. Washington, DC, American Psychiatric Association, 2000

Angelone SM, Bellini L, DiBella D, et al: Effects of fluvoxamine and citalopram in maintaining abstinence in a sample of Italian detoxified alcoholics. Alcohol Alcohol 33:151–156, 1998

Biederman J, Wilens T, Mick E, et al: Psychoactive substance use disorders in adults with attention deficit hyperactivity disorder (ADHD): effects of ADHD and psychiatric comorbidity. Am J Psychiatry 152:1652–1658, 1995

Bienvenu OJ, Samuels JF, Riddle MA, et al: The relationship of obsessive-compulsive disorder to possible spectrum disorders: results from a family study. Biol Psychiatry 48:287–293, 2000

Black DW, Moyer T: Clinical features and psychiatric comorbidity of subjects with pathological gambling behavior. Psychiatr Serv 49:1434–1439, 1998

Bland RC, Newman SC, Orn H, et al: Epidemiology of pathological gambling in Edmonton. Can J Psychiatry 38:108–112, 1993

Blaszczynski AP: Pathological gambling and obsessive-compulsive spectrum disorders. Psychol Rep 84:107–113, 1999

Blaszczynski AP, McConaghy N: SCL-90 assessed psychopathology in pathological gamblers. Psychol Rep 62:547–552, 1988

Blaszczynski AP, Steel Z, McConaghy N: Impulsivity in pathological gambling: the antisocial impulsivist. Addiction 92:75–87, 1997

Blum K, Sheridan PJ, Wood RC, et al: Dopamine D2 receptor gene variants: association and linkage studies in impulsive-addictive-compulsive behaviour. Pharmacogenetics 5:121–141, 1995

Carlton PL, Manowitz P: Physiological factors as determinants of pathological gambling. Journal of Gambling Behavior 3:274–285, 1988

Carlton PL, Manowitz P: Factors determining the severity of pathological gambling in males. J Gambl Stud 10:147–157, 1994

Carlton PL, Manowitz P, McBride H, et al: Attention deficit disorder and pathological gambling. J Clin Psychiatry 48:487–488, 1987

Cartwright C, DeCaria C, Hollander E: Pathological gambling: a clinical review. Practical Psychiatry and Behavioral Health 4:277–286, 1998

Castellani B, Rugle L: A comparison of pathological gamblers to alcoholics and cocaine misusers on impulsivity, sensation seeking, and craving. Int J Addict 30:275–289, 1995

Comings DE, Rosenthal RJ, Lesieur HR, et al: A study of the dopamine D2 receptor gene in pathological gambling. Pharmacogenetics 6:223–234, 1996

Cornelius JR, Salloum IM, Ehler JG, et al: Double-blind fluoxetine in depressed alcoholic smokers. Psychopharmacol Bull 33:165–170, 1997

Cunningham-Williams RM, Cottler LB, Compton WM III, et al: Taking chances: problem gamblers and mental health disorders—results from the St. Louis Epidemiologic Catchment Area Study. Am J Public Health 88:1093–1096, 1998

Cusack JR, Malaney KR, Depry DL: Insights about pathological gamblers: "chasing losses" in spite of the consequences. Postgrad Med 93:169–176, 1993

Daghestani AN, Elenz E, Crayton JW: Pathological gambling in hospitalized substance abusing veterans. J Clin Psychiatry 57:360–363, 1996

Dickerson MG: Gambling: a dependence without a drug. Int Rev Psychiatry 1:152–172, 1989

Foa EB, Franklin ME, Kozak MJ: Psychosocial treatments for obsessive-compulsive disorder: literature review, in Obsessive-Compulsive Disorder: Theory, Research and Treatment. Edited by Swinson RP, Antony MM, Rachman S, et al. New York, Guilford, 1998, pp 258–276

Grant JE, Kim SW: Comorbidity of impulse control disorders in pathological gamblers. Acta Psychiatr Scand 108:203–207, 2003

Haberman PW: Drinking and other self-indulgences: complements or counterattractions? Int J Addict 4:157–167, 1969

Haller R, Hinterhuber H: Treatment of pathological gambling with carbamazepine (case reports). Pharmacopsychiatry 27:129, 1994

Hantouche E, Merckaert P: Nosological classifications of obsessive-compulsive disorder (French). Ann Med Psychol (Paris) 149:393–408, 1991

Hoehn-Saric R, Barksdale VC: Impulsiveness in obsessive-compulsive patients. Br J Psychiatry 143:177–182, 1983

Hollander E, Skodol A, Oldham J (eds): Impulsivity and Compulsivity. Washington, DC, American Psychiatric Press, 1996

Hollander E, Stein DJ, Kwon JH, et al: Psychosocial function and economic costs of obsessive-compulsive disorder. CNS Spectr 2:16–25, 1997

Ibáñez A, de Castro IP, Fernandez-Piqueras J, et al: Pathological gambling and DNA polymorphic markers at MAO-A and MAO-B genes. Mol Psychiatry 5:105–109, 2000

Ibáñez A, Blanco C, Donahue E, et al: Psychiatric comorbidity in pathological gamblers seeking treatment. Am J Psychiatry 158:1733–1735, 2001

Kabel DI, Petty F: A placebo-controlled, double-blind study of fluoxetine in severe alcohol dependence: adjunctive pharmacotherapy during and after inpatient treatment. Alcohol Clin Exp Res 20:780–784, 1996

Kim SW, Grant JE: Personality dimensions in pathological gambling and obsessive-compulsive disorders. Psychiatry Res 104:205–212, 2001

Kranzler HR, Burleson JA, Korner P, et al: Placebo-controlled trial of fluoxetine as an adjunct to relapse prevention in alcoholics. Am J Psychiatry 152:391–397, 1995

Lesieur HR: The compulsive gambler's spiral of options and involvement. Psychiatry 42:79–87, 1979

Lesieur HR, Custer RL: Pathological gambling: roots, phases and treatment. Ann Am Acad Pol Soc Sci 474:146–156, 1984

Lesieur HR, Heineman M: Pathological gambling among youthful multiple substance abusers in a therapeutic community. Br J Addict 83:765–771, 1988

Lesieur HR, Blume SB, Zoppa RM: Alcoholism, drug abuse, and gambling. Alcohol Clin Exp Res 10:33–38, 1986

Linden RD, Pope HG Jr, Jonas JM: Pathological gambling and major affective disorder: preliminary findings. J Clin Psychiatry 47:201–203, 1986

Mannuzza S, Klein RG, Bessler A, et al: Adult outcome of hyperactive boys: educational achievement, occupational rank, and psychiatric status. Arch Gen Psychiatry 50:565–576, 1993

Marlatt GA, Gordon JR (eds): Relapse Prevention: Maintenance Strategies in the Treatment of Addictive Behaviors. New York, Guilford, 1985

McCormick RA, Russo AM, Ramirez LF, et al: Affective disorders among pathological gamblers seeking treatment. Am J Psychiatry 141:215–218, 1984

McCormick RA, Taber JI, Kruedelbach N, et al: Personality profiles of hospitalized pathological gamblers: the California Personality Inventory. J Clin Psychol 43:521–527, 1987

McElroy SL, Pope HG Jr, Keck PE Jr, et al: Are impulse-control disorders related to bipolar disorder? Compr Psychiatry 37:229–240, 1996

Moreno I, Saiz-Ruiz J, Lopez-Ibor JJ, et al: Ludopatia: un trastorno del animo? Anales de Psiquiatria 11:35–67, 1995

Moskowitz JA: Lithium and lady luck: use of lithium carbonate in compulsive gambling. N Y State J Med 80:785–788, 1980

Pallanti S, Baldini Rossi N, Sood E, et al: Nefazodone treatment of pathological gambling: a prospective open-label controlled trail. J Clin Psychiatry 63:1034–1039, 2002

Perez de Castro I, Ibáñez A, Saiz-Ruiz J, et al: Genetic contribution to pathological gambling: possible association between a functional DNA polymorphism at the serotonin transporter gene (5-HTT) and affected men. Pharmacogenetics 9:397–400, 1999

Petry NM: Pathological gamblers, with and without substance use disorders, discount delayed rewards at high rates. J Abnorm Psychol 110:482–487, 2001

Petry NM, Casarella T: Excessive discounting of delayed rewards in substance abusers with gambling problems. Drug Alcohol Depend 56:25–32, 1999

Petry NM, Kiluk BD: Suicidal ideation and suicide attempts in treatment-seeking pathological gamblers. J Nerv Ment Dis 190:462–469, 2002

Petry NM, Roll JM: A behavioral approach to understanding and treating pathological gambling. Semin Clin Neuropsychiatry 6:177–183, 2001

Pigott TA, Seay SM: A review of the efficacy of selective serotonin reuptake inhibitors in obsessive-compulsive disorder. J Clin Psychiatry 60:101–106, 1999

Potenza MN, Kosten TR, Rounsaville BJ: Pathological gambling. JAMA 286:141–144, 2001

Rasmussen SA, Eisen JL: The epidemiology and differential diagnosis of obsessive compulsive disorder. J Clin Psychiatry 53 (suppl):4–10, 1992

Rosselli M, Ardila A: Cognitive effects of cocaine and polydrug abuse. J Clin Exp Neuropsychol 18:122–135, 1996

Rugle L, Melamed L: Neuropsychological assessment of attention problems in pathological gamblers. J Nerv Ment Dis 181:107–112, 1993

Saiz-Ruiz J, Lopez-Ibor JJ: Gambling dependence: a severe form of self-destructive behavior. Paper presented at the 9th World Congress of Psychiatry, Vienna, June 6–12, 1993

Saiz-Ruiz J, Moreno I, Lopez-Ibor JJ: Pathological gambling: a clinical and therapeutic-evolutive study of a group of pathologic gamblers (Spanish). Actas Luso Esp Neurol Psiquiatr Cienc Afines 20:189–197, 1992

Specker SM, Carlson GA, Christenson GA, et al: Impulse control disorders and attention deficit disorder in pathological gamblers. Ann Clin Psychiatry 7:175–179, 1995

Spunt B, Lesieur H, Hunt D, et al: Gambling among methadone patients. Int J Addict 30:929–962, 1995

Steel Z, Blaszczynski A: Impulsivity, personality disorders and pathological gambling severity. Addiction 93:895–905, 1998

Stein DJ: Neurobiology of the obsessive-compulsive spectrum disorders. Biol Psychiatry 47:296–304, 2000

Stein DJ, Hollander E: Impulsive aggression and obsessive-compulsive disorder. Psychiatr Ann 23:389–395, 1993

Stein DJ, Hollander E, Simeon D, et al: Impulsivity scores in patients with obsessive-compulsive disorder. J Nerv Ment Dis 182:240–241, 1994

Sullivan S, Abbott M, McAvoy B, et al: Pathological gamblers: will they use a new telephone hotline? N Z Med J 107:313–315, 1994

Sylvain C, Ladouceur R, Boisvert JM: Cognitive and behavioral treatment of pathological gambling: a controlled study. J Consult Clin Psychol 65:727–732, 1997

Thorson JA, Powell FC, Hilt M: Epidemiology of gambling and depression in an adult sample. Psychol Rep 74:987–994, 1994

Volberg RA: The prevalence and demographics of pathological gamblers: implications for public health. Am J Public Health 84:237–241, 1994

Volberg RA: Gambling and Problem Gambling in New York: A 10-Year Replication Survey, 1986 to 1996. Albany, NY, New York Council on Problem Gambling, 1996

Warner LA, Kessler RC, Hughes M, et al: Prevalence and correlates of drug use and dependence in the United States. Arch Gen Psychiatry 52:219–229, 1995

World Health Organization: International Statistical Classification of Diseases and Related Health Problems, 10th Revision. Geneva, World Health Organization, 1992

Wray I, Phil M, Dickerson MG: Cessation of high frequency gambling and "withdrawal" symptoms. Br J Addict 76:401–405, 1981

Chapter 5

Adolescents and Young Adults

Randy Stinchfield, Ph.D., L.P.
Ken C. Winters, Ph.D.

To understand gambling among youths, it is important to first consider the context in which youth gambling occurs. There has been unprecedented growth in legalized gambling and a concomitant shift in public sentiment toward gambling. Although opinions vary about gambling, in general a negative sentiment toward gambling has shifted to one of tolerance and acceptance. In its public image, gambling has been transformed from an illegal vice to a legal and socially acceptable leisure activity for adults. The impact that these changes are having on youth populations is currently an important research topic.

Prevalence Studies

Three recent reviews of the prevalence of youth gambling concluded that although most youths have gambled, the majority do not experience adverse consequences or problems due to gambling (Jacobs 2000; National Research Council 1999; Shaffer et al. 1997). A small percentage of youths, however, exhibit serious gambling problems and meet criteria for pathological gambling. Between 3.2% and 8.4% of youths may have a serious gambling problem (past-year estimates) (Shaffer et al. 1997). The National Research Council (1999) reported that 52%–89% of youths have gambled in the past year. The National Research Council also reported past-year prevalence estimates for pathological gambling among adolescents of 6.1% (range, 0.3%–9.5%) and for pathological and problem gambling combined of 20%. From 1984 to 1999, gambling substantially increased among youths, with a parallel increase in the proportion of youths reporting gambling problems (Jacobs 2000). This increase in youth gambling may be due to the growth of the gambling industry and lotteries in particular and the increased social acceptance and promotion of gambling. Lotteries in particular may be culprits in the development of youth gambling because they are operated by state governments, are heavily advertised to the general public, and are widely available to youths (Jacobs 2000). Prevalence studies also indicate that youths tend to gamble informally—betting on games of personal skill, sports teams, and cards—until they come of legal age, at which time their preferences shift to legal forms of gambling. When legalized gambling is accessible to youths or the legal age is not enforced, youths are more likely to participate in legalized gambling (Wynne et al. 1996).

The National Research Council (1999) reported that adolescent rates of pathological gambling could be more than three times those for adults, although the report acknowledges that the rates of adolescent pathological gambling may not be directly comparable to adult rates due to differences in instruments and definitions between these two groups of studies. Even within youth studies, it is difficult to make direct comparisons between results due to the differences in measurement instruments, definitions, and cutoff scores across studies.

Recent North American youth gambling surveys have been conducted in Alberta, Louisiana, New York, and Oregon; a U.S. national study was also conducted. An Alberta survey conducted in 1995 (Wynne et al. 1996) used the South Oaks Gambling Screen (SOGS) (Lesieur and Blume 1987). This study was a telephone survey of 972 youths between ages 12 and 17. It was found that 651 youths (67% of the sample) gambled; 8% were identified as problem gamblers (using the SOGS and a cutoff score of 5 or more); and 15% were at risk of developing a gambling problem (SOGS score of 3 or 4). This study suggested that there are "problem gambling social groups"; that is, a group of young males who have gambling as their primary pastime.

This study found higher reported rates of problem gambling among Alberta youths compared with adults (Wynne et al. 1994; Wynne Resources 1998). Youths were four times more likely to be at risk or to be problem gamblers than adults (23% of youths vs. 5% of adults). The authors offered the following possible explanations for the particularly high prevalence estimates of problem gambling in Alberta youths: 1) Alberta has more forms of licensed gambling and has had them longer than other Canadian provinces and the United States; 2) gambling vendors do not routinely ask for proof of age; 3) the message from gambling advertising suggests that gambling is a harmless amusement; 4) many youth programs are funded by forms of gambling (e.g., bingo and raffles) for which the youths sell and purchase tickets; and 5) Alberta society at large does not appear concerned about gambling among youths. Although the authors of the survey accept these rates at face value, it may be that the rates reflect response bias such as overreporting, as has been reported by others (e.g., Ladouceur et al. 2000).

A survey of the gambling behavior of 12,066 Louisiana school students in grades 6–12 during the 1996–1997 school year found that 86% of the sample had gambled in their lifetime (Westphal et al. 2000). However, the majority gambled infrequently; that is, monthly or less often. Findings on frequent gambling (i.e., weekly or more often) were as follows: 16.5% gambled on instant scratch-off lottery tickets, 12.5% made sports bets, 10.5% bet on cards, 10% wagered on games of personal skill, and 9% gambled on the lottery by picking numbers. Problem gambling was measured with the South Oaks Gambling Screen–Revised for Adolescents (SOGS-RA) (Winters et al. 1993b), using a cutoff score of 4, and the prevalence estimate was reported as 6%.

A telephone survey of 1,103 New York adolescents ages 13–17 conducted in 1997 found that 75% had gambled in the past year and that 15% had gambled weekly or more often (Volberg 1998). There were differences between boys and girls: 80% of boys and 70% of girls had gambled in the past year; and 23% of boys and 7% of girls had gambled weekly or more often in the past year. Lottery gambling was related to age, with 20% of 13-year-olds and 36% of 17-year-olds gambling on the lottery in the past year. Only 26 respondents (2% of the sample) had gambled in a casino in the past year. The rate of problem gambling was 2.4%.

Carlson and Moore (1998) surveyed 1,000 youths ages 13–17 in Oregon in 1998 via a telephone interview and found that 66% had gambled for money in the past year. Survey respondents were administered the SOGS-RA to measure problem gambling, and 4.1% received a score of 4 or more and were therefore classified as having a gambling problem.

Wiebe (1999) recruited 1,000 youths in Manitoba for a survey. This study used the SOGS-RA to measure problem gambling and found that 78% of the sample had gambled in the past year and that 3% exhibited problem gambling (i.e., SOGS-RA score of 4 or more). This survey is one of the few that asked youths about Internet gambling. Because youths are facile with computers and because the Internet has a degree of anonymity (i.e., an underage user can pose as an adult), there is significant concern that youths may become involved in Internet gambling. However, this study showed that of all forms of gambling, Internet gambling was engaged in the least frequently, possibly because many youths do not have credit cards, a requirement for Internet gambling.

A U.S. national survey of 534 youths ages 16–17 was conducted in 1998 by the National Opinion Research Center (NORC) via a randomized telephone survey (National Opinion Research Center 1999). The NORC used DSM-IV (American Psychiatric Association 1994) diagnostic criteria to measure problem and pathological gambling. The NORC found that 67% had gambled and that 3% were classified as problem or pathological gamblers (i.e., three or more DSM-IV criteria endorsed). Unfortunately, the NORC did not report a separate number for pathological gamblers due to the small sample. This study has two methodological considerations that need to be acknowledged in interpreting the results. First, this study employed an improved measurement instrument, that is, DSM-IV diagnostic criteria, rather than the typical set of screening items. Second, this study was intended to be a national survey; however, the sample size of 500 is smaller than most state and provincial surveys.

Four studies provided information about changes in youth gambling over time. The first study had a longitudinal design whereby 702 Minnesota adolescents were surveyed by telephone in 1990 (at the onset of the Minnesota Lottery), and 532 participants from the original sample (76% response rate) were resurveyed 1 year later (Winters et al. 1995). The investigators reported that rates of gambling and problem gambling did not change in this sample. Instead, patterns of gambling changed, with a shift away from informal betting to legalized forms of gambling, particularly among youths who reached the legal age for gambling (age 18) during the course of the follow-up interval.

The second study, conducted in Texas, involved a telephone survey administered in different years to two separate samples from the same general population of Texas youths (Wallisch 1993, 1996). The survey was first administered in 1992 to 924 adolescents and was later administered to a new sample of 3,079 youths in 1995. Wallisch found that gambling rates remained relatively stable from 1992 to 1995, with rates of gambling in the past year remaining at 67% and weekly gambling dropping slightly from 14% in 1992 to 11% in 1995. Rates of problem gambling also declined from 5% in 1992 to 2.3% in 1995.

The third study was conducted in the state of Washington by Volberg and Moore (1999). This study compared a 1993 telephone survey of 1,045 Washington youths to a second telephone survey of 1,000 youths in 1999. The surveys were administered to two separate, randomly selected samples drawn from the Washington population of youths between ages 13 and 17. The investigators found an increase in nongamblers from 16.7% to 22.4% and a decrease in weekly gamblers from 9.6% to 7.7%. The prevalence rate of problem gambling remained stable at 1% for both surveys.

In the fourth study, three waves of Minnesota Student Survey data—collected from almost the entire population of ninth- and twelfth-grade Minnesota public school students in 1992, 1995, and 1998—were examined (Stinchfield 2001). The 1992 sample included a total of 122,700 sixth-, ninth-, and twelfth-grade public school students. Gambling items were not administered to the sixth graders in the 1995 and 1998 surveys due to the need for a brief survey for sixth-grade students. The 1995 sample included a total of 75,900 ninth- and twelfth-grade students, and the 1998 sample included a total of 78,582 ninth- and twelfth-grade students. There were five gambling activity items and two gambling problem items. This set of three Minnesota studies allowed for two different types of examination of change over time. First, the same class or cohort of youths can be studied as they mature. This study demonstrated that a higher percentage of boys than girls were involved in frequent gambling and that this percentage increased with age. Also, the percentages of weekly and daily gamblers among twelfth-grade boys and girls and ninth-grade boys increased in 1998.

In summary, it appears that the frequency of gambling among youths has for the most part remained stable, and that according to some studies it has declined in the general population. However, participation in legalized gambling among youths who reach age 18 appears to be increasing, and the number of older youths, particularly males, who gamble at a weekly or daily rate also seems to be increasing. Thus, for most youths the rate of gambling participation is remaining about the same or is decreasing, but for a small percentage of youths it is increasing. Although the finding that gambling has not increased for most youths is encouraging, there is continued concern about the small group of youths who have increased their gambling. It will be important to continue to monitor the gambling behavior of youths over time.

Assessment of Youth Gambling

How is problem gambling best defined and measured? The increasingly accepted standard for defining problem gambling is by the diagnostic criteria of DSM-IV-TR (American Psychiatric Association 2000) (see Appendix A). The SOGS was originally based on DSM-III (American

Psychiatric Association 1980) diagnostic criteria for pathological gambling (Lesieur and Blume 1987). Since that time, other instruments have been developed that assess each diagnostic criterion from DSM-IV-TR. (One example is Fisher's [2000] revised version of her DSM-IV-TR–based instrument for assessing pathological gambling in juveniles, the DSM-IV Multiple Response–Juvenile, or DSM-IV-MR-J.) Pathological gambling is diagnosed by summing the set of 10 DSM-IV-TR criteria. A cutoff score of 5 out of 10 is the current standard; however, some research suggests that a cutoff score of 4 maximizes classification accuracy and minimizes classification errors for adults (Stinchfield 2003).

When measuring problem gambling among youths, investigators generally use more liberal cutoff scores than they use with adults. These lower cutoff scores have typically been used to identify more individuals showing early signs of problem gambling. For example, Winters and colleagues (1993b) used a cutoff score of 4 in the SOGS-RA rather than the standard SOGS cutoff score of 5 used with adults. In the DSM-IV-MR-J, Fisher (2000) also used a cutoff score of 4 rather than 5. This practice has continued without adequate classification accuracy research to validate this lowered cutoff score.

The fact that problem gambling among youths has been measured using different definitions, different instruments, different time frames, and different cutoff scores raises the question of whether prevalence rates can be compared within and across age groups. For example, in a meta-analysis by Shaffer et al. (1997), a prevalence rate for youth problem gambling of 5.8% was computed, with a 95% confidence interval of 3.2%–8.4%. However, many of the studies included in the meta-analysis employed quite divergent methodologies for classifying problem gamblers. Studies used different instruments, including the SOGS, the SOGS-RA, the Massachusetts Gambling Screen (Shaffer et al. 1994), and DSM-based questionnaires, and some studies that used the same instrument used different cutoff scores and different time frames (e.g., past-year vs. lifetime gambling).

Gender Differences

Among the most consistent and robust findings across studies of youth gambling are that boys are more involved in gambling than are girls and that boys also have higher rates of problem gambling than girls (e.g., Gupta and Derevensky 1998a; Stinchfield 2001; Wallisch 1993; Wynne et al. 1996). More boys than girls gamble, and boys gamble more frequently than girls. Boys spend more money and more time gambling than girls. Boys wager on a greater variety of forms of gambling than do girls. However, girls may catch up to boys in gambling, as they have done in the use of tobacco, alcohol, and other drugs. Boys and girls also have different gambling preferences. Boys tend to bet on games of personal skill such as golf or billiards and on lotteries, card games, and sports teams. Girls, if they gamble, most frequently bet on lotteries and sports teams (Stinchfield 2001; Stinchfield et al. 1997; Winters et al. 1993a). Another consistent finding across studies is that older youths (ages 14–18 years) gamble more often than younger youths (age 13 or younger) (e.g., Arcuri et al. 1985; Stinchfield 2000).

Comparison to Adult Gamblers

Prevalence rates of pathological gambling are higher among youths than among adults (e.g., Jacobs 2000; National Research Council 1999; Shaffer and Hall 1996). Past-year estimates for serious gambling problems among youths range from 3.2% to 8.4% (Shaffer et al. 1997). In comparison, prevalence rates of pathological gambling in adults are between 1% and 3% (American Psychiatric Association 1994). Both Shaffer et al. (1997) and the National Research Council (1999) reported youth rates for pathological gambling about three times the rates for adults.

Evidence suggests that these high youth rates may not be accurate. For most other addictions, such as alcohol and drug abuse, youths do not have rates three times those of adults. Similarly, youths do not call gambling help lines or hotlines three times more frequently than adults, nor are there three times as many youths than adults coming for treatment. In fact, few youths call gambling help lines and even fewer come for treatment. There are at least four possible explanations for this discrepancy in youth and adult rates. First, the reported youth rates are accurate and there are in fact two or more times as many adolescent pathological gamblers as there are adult pathological gamblers. Second, the youth rates are not accurate due to a lack of consistency in methodology, definitions, measurement, cutoff scores, and diagnostic criteria across studies—particularly the use of lower cutoff scores for youths in some studies. The practice of using a lower cutoff score for youths has the effect of increasing the number of individuals identified with a gambling problem and is likely to account in part for the higher prevalence rates reported for youth problem gambling. Third, the rates are not accurate due to youths exaggerating their involvement in gambling. Fourth, the rates are not accurate due to measurement error resulting from the use of adult instruments that are not appropriate for youths (e.g., Ladouceur et al. 2000) to assess problem gambling among youths. Data support the notion that the SOGS and SOGS-RA, the most commonly used measures of problem gambling, tend to overestimate rates of problem and pathological gambling—that is, they err on the side of false-positive results (Derevensky and Gupta 2000; Stinchfield 2002). This type of error is acceptable for a screening instrument, but it highlights limitations of the use of the instrument for estimating prevalence.

It does not appear that a separate set of criteria is necessary for youths. Pathological gambling is not a strictly adolescent disorder, nor does there appear to be a unique adolescent version of the disorder. However, it may be necessary to adapt some diagnostic criteria to take into account the developmental stage of adolescents.

Association With Other Behaviors

Several studies have identified correlates of gambling and problem gambling among youths. Gupta and Derevensky (1998a, 1998b) found that use of tobacco, alcohol, and drugs was related to the severity of gambling problems. In two consecutive telephone surveys of Texas youths in 1992 and 1995, Wallisch (1996) found that problem gamblers were more likely to be male, to be younger, to be from a minority racial or ethnic group, to work 10 or more hours per week, to have a weekly income of $10 or more, to have favorable attitudes toward gambling, to expect to make money at gambling, and to have parents who gambled. The youth study in Alberta found that youths with a gambling problem were more likely to be in trouble with the police; to feel that they could not confide in parents, teachers, school counselors, and ministers; to feel ignored or rejected by their family; to report negative school experiences; to have started gambling early (often before age 10); to report that their family members gambled; to wager large amounts of money; to borrow money for gambling; to steal or sell personal property; to report feeling anxious, worried, upset, or depressed; to smoke cigarettes; and to frequently drink alcohol and use illicit drugs. This study suggests that problem gamblers begin gambling early in life; consider gambling part of their family norm; have not had success in school; feel alienated from their family and community; use tobacco, alcohol, and other drugs; have a negative affect; and behave antisocially. Together, the findings of these studies suggest that the typical youthful problem gambler is a fairly troubled individual and that excessive gambling is part of a larger constellation of psychological distress, family dysfunction, and deviant behavior (Wynne et al. 1996).

In a telephone survey of gambling among 702 youths in the general population of Minnesota, youths with greater gambling involvement were more likely to be male, to use drugs regularly, to have parents who gambled, to report a history of delinquency, and to demonstrate poor academic achievement (Winters et al. 1993a). In the Minnesota Student

Survey, variables associated with gambling frequency included antisocial behavior, male gender, alcohol use, tobacco use, age, feeling bad about the amount of money gambled, a desire to stop gambling, and sexual behavior (Stinchfield 2000). Volberg (1993) conducted a telephone survey of 1,054 Washington State adolescents and found that use of tobacco, alcohol, and drugs was associated with gambling frequency and problem gambling. These studies indicate that gambling may be part of a constellation of deviant behaviors that are mainly exhibited by males, including frequent alcohol use, tobacco use, drug use, physical violence, vandalism, shoplifting, and truancy. These risky behaviors may play a role in the development or maintenance of gambling behavior and problem gambling.

The 1992 Minnesota Student Survey data show concurrent rates of gambling and other risky behaviors for sixth-, ninth-, and twelfth-grade public school students. Frequent gambling was more prevalent among sixth graders, particularly boys, than was frequent tobacco, alcohol, or marijuana use. However, as boys aged, more of them reported frequent tobacco and alcohol use, and by the time of the twelfth grade, frequent tobacco use and alcohol use were equal in prevalence to frequent gambling. Frequent gambling appears at an early age in boys and appears to precede frequent tobacco and alcohol use. For a small percentage of girls (5%), frequent gambling also appears at an early age but is superseded by frequent tobacco and alcohol use when the girls reach ninth grade and is relatively infrequent by the twelfth grade compared with tobacco use. In other words, frequent gambling begins early for boys and remains a common risky behavior through ninth and twelfth grades, whereas only a small percentage of girls are involved in frequent gambling, and by the ninth and twelfth grades gambling is overshadowed by frequent tobacco and alcohol use.

In summary, excessive gambling seems to go hand in hand with other high-risk behaviors such as use of tobacco, alcohol, and other drugs during adolescence, and gambling appears to precede other risky behaviors and is often initiated during the preadolescent years. These findings suggest that there is a small segment of the youth population—predominantly males—who are involved in a number of high-risk behaviors (gambling being one) and that any prevention efforts may need to address the constellation of high-risk behaviors rather than focusing on gambling alone.

Future Research

Most research to date has focused on the basic questions of the extent of youth gambling and the prevalence of problem gambling among youth populations. The field should begin to address more specific empirical questions about the origin, etiology, and correlates of problem gambling. A pressing research question is whether youth gambling will increase over time. The trend from the few longitudinal studies conducted so far indicates that most youth gambling has remained fairly stable. However, it will be important to continue to monitor youth gambling over longer periods of time, particularly given temporal changes in societal acceptance and availability of legalized forms of gambling.

A second basic question for future research is why youths gamble. Little is known about how youth problem gambling begins, what variables maintain problem gambling, how and why youths move from social and recreational gambling to problem gambling, and which youths are most likely to become problem gamblers. Youths gamble for different reasons, and it will be important to develop a model of the onset and maintenance of youth gambling that will provide a scientific basis for the development of prevention and intervention programs. Improved identification of problem gambling at early stages would significantly facilitate prevention and intervention efforts. Multiple correlates of youth problem gambling have been identified, including antisocial behavior and use of tobacco, alcohol, and drugs. However, the extent to which specific characteristics have a causal relationship to gambling and problem gambling is still being investigated. Longitudinal studies need to be conducted to address the question of causality and the order of onset of different problem behaviors (Lesieur 1989).

The finding that youths have higher rates of problem and pathological gambling compared with adults demands attention. It will be important to examine the extent to which this finding reflects a true rate of adolescent pathological gambling or a measurement artifact. It will also be important to develop screening and assessment instruments specifically for youths that take developmental issues into consideration.

Along with legalization and expansion of gambling, the public is exposed to daily gambling advertising in multiple media. A question arises: What effect does gambling advertising have on youths? Gambling advertisements frequently encourage gambling with the message that it is a quick and easy way to get rich. Advertisements generally do not contain warnings about possible adverse consequences of gambling such as the effects of financial losses. Youths may not fully understand the relative probabilities of winning and losing and therefore may be susceptible to promotions suggesting rapid and easy financial gains.

A new and understudied form of gambling that may pose a particular risk for youths is Internet gambling. Youths are generally quite adept with computers and the Internet. The Internet has gambling sites that provide online casino-style gambling, including blackjack, poker, slots, and roulette. These sites require the user to pay for gambling with a credit card. Because a computer or Internet site cannot determine who is operating the computer, youths can readily access Internet gambling sites. Internet gambling is more accessible to youths than casinos or other gambling venues and is virtually unregulated at this time. Internet gambling by youths is currently relatively unexplored, and, given the recent growth of the Internet gambling industry, it will be important to investigate the impact on youths of this potentially high-risk form of gambling.

Conclusion

Most studies report that youths have gambled on legalized games. Underage gambling is largely illegal and is potentially harmful for youths. The extent of underage gambling needs to be examined more closely, and an investigation into how underage youths gain access to forms of gambling that are legal for adults is warranted. Next, plans targeting both vendors and youths should be developed and implemented to prevent youths from accessing these forms of gambling. Current data indicating that most youths gamble infrequently suggest that prevention efforts aimed at a general adolescent population should include an educational message about the probabilities of winning and the risks associated with gambling. However, data showing that some youths appear to be increasing their involvement in gambling suggest that tailored, multifaceted prevention and intervention approaches will be important (Dickson et al. 2002). For most youths, informal gambling is an infrequent and harmless pastime. However, the risk exists that informal gambling will develop into problem and pathological gambling, and therefore youths need to receive accurate information about the inherent risks of gambling and appropriate protection (through prevention and treatment efforts) from gambling problems.

References

American Psychiatric Association: Diagnostic and Statistical Manual of Mental Disorders, 3rd Edition. Washington, DC, American Psychiatric Association, 1980

American Psychiatric Association: Diagnostic and Statistical Manual of Mental Disorders, 4th Edition. Washington, DC, American Psychiatric Association, 1994

American Psychiatric Association: Diagnostic and Statistical Manual of Mental Disorders, 4th Edition, Text Revision. Washington, DC, American Psychiatric Association, 2000

Arcuri AF, Lester D, Smith FO: Shaping adolescent gambling behavior. Adolescence 20:935–938, 1985

Carlson MJ, Moore TL: Adolescent Gambling in Oregon: A Report to the Oregon Gambling Addiction Treatment Foundation. Salem, OR, Oregon Gambling Addiction Treatment Foundation, 1998

Derevensky JL, Gupta R: Prevalence estimates of adolescent gambling: a comparison of the SOGS-RA, DSM-IV-J, and the GA 20 Questions. J Gambl Stud 16:227–251, 2000

Dickson LM, Derevensky JL, Gupta R: The prevention of gambling problems in youth: a conceptual framework. J Gambl Stud 18:97–159, 2002

Fisher S: Developing the DSM-IV-DSM-IV criteria to identify adolescent problem gambling in non-clinical populations. J Gambl Stud 16:253–273, 2000

Gupta R, Derevensky JL: Adolescent gambling behavior: a prevalence study and examination of the correlates associated with problem gambling. J Gambl Stud 14:319–345, 1998a

Gupta R, Derevensky JL: An empirical examination of Jacobs' General Theory of Addictions: do adolescent gamblers fit the theory? J Gambl Stud 14:17–49, 1998b

Jacobs DF: Juvenile gambling in North America: an analysis of long term trends and future prospects. J Gambl Stud 16:119–152, 2000

Ladouceur R, Bouchard C, Rheaume N, et al: Is the SOGS an accurate measure of pathological gambling among children, adolescents and adults? J Gambl Stud 16:1–24, 2000

Lesieur HR: Current research in pathological gambling and gaps in the literature, in Compulsive Gambling: Theory, Research, and Practice. Edited by Shaffer HJ, Stein SA, Gambino B, et al. Lexington, MA, Lexington Books, 1989, pp 225–248

Lesieur HR, Blume SB: The South Oaks Gambling Screen (SOGS): a new instrument for the identification of pathological gamblers. Am J Psychiatry 144:1184–1188, 1987

National Opinion Research Center: Gambling Impact and Behavior Study: Report to the National Gambling Impact Study Commission. Chicago, IL, National Opinion Research Center at the University of Chicago, 1999. Available at: http://www.norc.uchicago.edu/new/gamb-fin.htm. Accessed December 13, 2003.

National Research Council: Pathological Gambling: A Critical Review. Washington, DC, National Academy Press, 1999

Shaffer HJ, Hall MN: Estimating the prevalence of adolescent gambling disorders: a quantitative synthesis and guide toward standard gambling nomenclature. J Gambl Stud 12:193–214, 1996

Shaffer HJ, LaBrie R, Scanlan KM, et al: Pathological gambling among adolescents: Massachusetts Gambling Screen (MAGS). J Gambl Stud 10:339–362, 1994

Shaffer HJ, Hall MN, Vander Bilt J: Estimating the Prevalence of Disordered Gambling Behavior in the United States and Canada: A Meta-Analysis. Boston, MA, Harvard Medical School, Division on Addictions, 1997

Stinchfield R: Gambling and correlates of gambling among Minnesota public school students. J Gambl Stud 16:153–173, 2000

Stinchfield R: A comparison of gambling among Minnesota public school students in 1992, 1995 and 1998. J Gambl Stud 17:273–296, 2001

Stinchfield R: Reliability, validity, and classification accuracy of the South Oaks Gambling Screen (SOGS). Addict Behav 27:1–19, 2002

Stinchfield R: Reliability, validity, and classification accuracy of a measure of DSM-IV diagnostic criteria for pathological gambling. Am J Psychiatry 160:180–182, 2003

Stinchfield R, Cassuto N, Winters K, et al: Prevalence of gambling among Minnesota public school students in 1992 and 1995. J Gambl Stud 13:25–48, 1997

Volberg R: Gambling and Problem Gambling Among Adolescents in Washington State. Albany, NY, Gemini Research, 1993

Volberg R: Gambling and Problem Gambling Among Adolescents in New York. Albany, NY, New York Council on Problem Gambling, 1998

Volberg R, Moore WL: Gambling and Problem Gambling Among Adolescents in Washington State: A Replication Study, 1993 to 1999. Report to the Washington State Lottery. Northampton, MA, Gemini Research, 1999

Wallisch L: Gambling in Texas: 1992 Texas Survey of Adolescent Gambling Behavior. Austin, TX, Texas Commission on Alcohol and Drug Abuse, 1993

Wallisch L: Gambling in Texas: 1995 Surveys of Adult and Adolescent Gambling Behavior. Austin, TX, Texas Commission on Alcohol and Drug Abuse, 1996

Westphal JR, Rush JA, Stevens L, et al: Gambling behavior of Louisiana students in grades 6 through 12. Psychiatr Serv 51:96–99, 2000

Wiebe J: Manitoba Youth Gambling Prevalence Study. Winnipeg, MB, Awareness and Information, Addictions Foundation of Manitoba, 1999

Winters KC, Stinchfield R, Fulkerson J: Patterns and characteristics of adolescent gambling. J Gambl Stud 9:371–386, 1993a

Winters KC, Stinchfield R, Fulkerson J: Toward the development of an adolescent gambling problem severity scale. J Gambl Stud 9:63–84, 1993b

Winters KC, Stinchfield R, Kim L: Monitoring adolescent gambling in Minnesota. J Gambl Stud 11:165–183, 1995

Wynne H, Smith G, Volberg R: Gambling and Problem Gambling in Alberta. Edmonton, AB, Canada, Alberta Lotteries and Gaming, 1994

Wynne HJ, Smith GJ, Jacobs DF: Adolescent Gambling and Problem Gambling in Alberta. Report prepared for the Alberta Alcohol and Drug Abuse Commission. Edmonton, AB, Canada, Wynne Resources, 1996

Wynne Resources: Adult Gambling and Problem Gambling in Alberta, 1998. Edmonton, AB, Canada, Alberta Alcohol and Drug Abuse Commission, 1998

Chapter 6

Older Adults

Rani A. Desai, M.P.H., Ph.D.

Adults over age 65 represent a large and growing demographic in the U.S. population and arguably a key target market for the gambling industry. However, relatively little is known about the effects of gambling on older adults. This chapter begins with a review of what is known about the prevalence of and risk factors for problem and pathological gambling in the elderly. Next, the relatively sparse data on the health effects of gambling on the elderly are described. Finally, treatment issues that may differ between older versus younger adults (or that may be unique to older adults) with problem and pathological gambling are explored.

Problem and Pathological Gambling

Prevalence Estimates

Arguably the best data on the relationship between age and problem or pathological gambling come from the Gambling Impact and Behavior Study (GIBS) (National Opinion Research Center 1999). This national study divided subjects into five categories: those who had not gambled ("nongamblers"), those who had gambled and had experienced none of the DSM-IV (American Psychiatric Association 1994) symptoms of problem and pathological gambling ("low-risk" gamblers), those who had experienced one or two symptoms ("at-risk" gamblers), those who experienced three or four symptoms ("problem" gamblers), and those who had experienced five or more symptoms ("pathological" gamblers). Increased mental health and psychosocial problems were associated with increased severity of gambling (National Opinion Research Center 1999). In general, prevalence rates for disordered gambling decrease as age increases. Those over age 65 have the lowest rates of pathological gambling (0.2% vs. 0.3%–0.9% for younger age groups); among the lowest rates of problem gambling (0.6% vs. 1.0% among those ages 18–29); and the lowest rates of at-risk gambling (1.7% vs. 2.1%–3.9% in younger age groups).

Phenomenology

Problem and pathological gamblers experience many of the same symptoms as people with other addictions: they experience tolerance (needing to gamble more for the same effect), symptoms of withdrawal, and loss of control over the addictive behavior. This pattern has been demonstrated among gamblers of all ages.

> Bill and Sue were a retired couple living on Long Island, with their one surviving child living in upstate New York and few surviving friends in their neighborhood. They had worked several jobs each throughout most of their lives, and they found retirement to be boring. These feelings were exacerbated by the fact that Sue was confined to a wheelchair with both circulatory and cardiovascular conditions, making it difficult to find leisure activities that were both accessible and enjoyable for both of them.
>
> An acquaintance suggested that they join a group going to Atlantic City, and the couple decided to go. They spent an enjoyable weekend, winning over $500 between them, and decided to make such a trip a more regular part of their routine. Within a few months they were going nearly once a week and had added daily lotto play to their gambling routines.
>
> Within a year, they were gambling almost continuously. They were rarely at home and spent most of their time on the road, traveling up and down the eastern seaboard to various casinos from Connecticut to Florida. Their conversations with family were almost exclusively centered on recent wins and "near wins," the prizes they had won from casinos for being such good customers, and their wish to own a mobile home so that they would not have to pay for hotel rooms.
>
> A "crisis" ensued when Sue had to be hospitalized for surgery and remained in the hospital to recover. After a few days, both Bill and Sue became very restless, talked of nothing else except going to the casino, bought large numbers of daily lotto tickets, and spent hours strategizing their lottery number picks. After a week, Sue left the hospital, and despite doctor recommendations to rest at home, they immediately embarked on another casino trip.

During this time the couple had neglected their home and their home insurance. When an electrical fire resulted in the destruction of their home, they were unable to recoup losses. Sue died a few days later of an apparent heart attack, possibly related to the stress of losing their home. With no home and virtually no financial assets, Bill subsequently moved to Georgia to live with his brother. He continues to gamble occasionally, although he says that the "fun is gone out of it." He spends most of his time helping his brother in a contracting business and playing in a country-western band.

It has been suggested that the development of problem gambling follows a predictable course. This course, described by Custer (1984), begins with a winning phase, progresses to a losing phase, and ends with a desperation phase, which continues either indefinitely or until extreme events force a change in gambling behavior. Little indicates that the course is substantially different among the elderly (Custer 1984), although some manifestations of gambling difficulties may be different in the elderly, such as sources of income, spending behaviors, borrowing behaviors, and engagement in criminal behavior.

The financial repercussions of problem gambling may differ for the elderly. Older adults are more likely to be retired and thus to be surviving on annuity income (e.g., Social Security, pensions), savings, and investment income. Elderly gamblers are less likely to have employment income, a fact that may either change patterns of spending on gambling or change the impact of that spending. Older adults with no employment income have more difficulty recovering from financial losses and may be more likely than younger gamblers to exhaust savings, cash in investments, and spend annuity income (Desai et al., in press; Pavalko 2002). The amount of money spent by a younger, working individual may have less overall impact than the same amount spent by a retired gambler with limited ability to recover from a loss.

Although the effects of financial losses may be more pronounced in the elderly, the effects of gambling on work and family relationships may appear less pronounced. Difficulties related to either work or family relationships, which are symptoms included in the DSM diagnosis of pathological gambling, may be less relevant for older adults who are retired and may be widowed. For example, retired gamblers are less likely to commit work-related white-collar crimes (e.g., embezzlement) to obtain gambling money. Similarly, they may have fewer family members than younger gamblers from whom to borrow money to continue gambling. Because there may be less opportunity to engage in certain behaviors that constitute symptoms of pathological gambling, the impact of gambling on these aspects of life for older adults may be underestimated.

Unique Triggers and Risk Factors for Pathological Gambling

A number of risk factors for the onset of problem and pathological gambling have been identified, and some of these risk factors may be either stronger or entirely unique for older adults. These include gambling opportunities and the marketing practices of the gambling industry, social isolation, depression and anxiety, and biological changes that are associated with both older age and gambling behavior.

> Anna, a 67-year-old woman, was in excellent health until the death of her husband of 40 years. After her husband's death, she became very depressed and withdrawn. Having never held a full-time job after her marriage, she had difficulty filling her time now that she no longer was cooking and cleaning for her husband. In addition, she had very little understanding of her financial assets. After several falls, she moved to a supportive-care housing unit, paid for by life insurance and other savings set aside by her husband.
>
> Anna's mood improved after the move, partially because she had a network of friends and a regular schedule of social activities, including bingo games. She and a small group of friends would play bingo several times a week, traveling to various sites for games on different nights. Although she never spent very much at any one time, Anna's financial assets were quite small and were taxed by the costs of her housing. She began to respond to mail solicitations for credit cards, taking cash advances to finance her gambling that she was unable to pay back. She also regularly asked her children for cash sums to gamble, saying that she needed money for medications or unexpected expenses.
>
> Becoming suspicious of these increasingly frequent requests, her son investigated and found that his mother was gambling and losing about $100 a week playing bingo. Since this was a substantial portion of her disposable income, and since she was in a substantial amount of debt due to her cash advances, the son became very concerned. When confronted, Anna angrily objected to being treated like a child, and she accused her son of wanting to get her money. Initially refusing to seek treatment, Anna cut off contact with her son. After her lease at the supported housing community was terminated due to her inability to pay the rent, she agreed to attend Gamblers Anonymous meetings. She subsequently got treatment for both her gambling problem and her depression, allowed her son to manage her money, reduced and eventually eliminated her credit card debt with the help of a debt counselor, and rebuilt a network of social ties around nongambling activities.

Research has consistently shown that opportunity plays an important role in the prevalence of gambling, and by extension the prevalence of problem and pathological gambling. The increased availability of state-sponsored lotteries and the proliferation of casinos have affected people of all ages. Because older adult retirees have more disposable time to engage in gambling behavior, however, their opportunities to gamble have increased markedly (McNeilly and Burke 2002). In addition, states that have high numbers of retired citizens (e.g., Florida, Arizona) have seen increases in the availability of gambling activities, and many such venues have incentive programs specifically targeting elders (e.g., free bus rides, discounted meals). Finally, many extended-care facilities offer gambling activities (e.g., bingo games for money or casino day trips) as a means of social interaction and activity. This increased opportunity to gamble may place older people at greater risk for development of gambling-related problems.

As adults age, they often experience the loss of traditional social roles associated with being parents, having employment, and even being in a marriage (McNeilly and Burke 2002; Pavalko 2002). The loss of such roles, along with the increased likelihood that children will not live in close proximity, can lead to feelings of social isolation, boredom, and even depression and anxiety. These feelings may in turn place the elderly at increased risk for developing gambling problems. Gambling activities may help to alleviate these feelings by providing entertaining sensory stimulation, a chance to socialize, and a chance to escape from everyday problems and feelings (McNeilly and Burke 2000, 2001, 2002; Pavalko 2002), although no direct evidence shows that geriatric depression leads to gambling (Grant et al. 2001).

In addition, although elderly people may find themselves restricted in the types of physical activities they can engage in (e.g., due to physical or mental decline), gambling venues are handicap accessible, and many forms of gambling (e.g., slot machines) are relatively passive forms of entertainment requiring little cognitive ability (McNeilly and Burke 2002). This ease of accessibility is cause for some concern, particularly because slot machines appear to be a favorite of older casino gamblers (Grant et al. 2001), and some research has shown that progression to addiction is particularly fast among slot machine players (Breen and Zimmerman 2002).

A final possible risk factor that is relatively unique to elderly patients—but that requires much more study—is the cognitive and physical decline associated with diseases such as Parkinson's disease and dementia. Several case reports have highlighted patients being treated for Parkinson's disease who developed gambling addictions concurrent with the start of pro-dopaminergic therapies (Gschwandtner et al. 2001; Molina et al. 2000; Seedat et al. 2000). Changes in brain neurobiology associated with normal aging, which are implicated in addictive behaviors, may be one explanation for the reduction of gambling behaviors in older versus younger adults. Gambling may also enhance dopaminergic function in older adults and may thus be more strongly reinforced in older adults who have naturally diminishing dopamine levels. The extent to which dopaminergic function is associated with problem and pathological gambling across the life span warrants direct investigation.

It is unlikely that individuals with advanced forms of dementia are capable of engaging in gambling. However, early forms of dementia and other forms of cognitive decline may place older adults at greater risk for gambling-related problems by reducing their ability to weigh risks, impairing memory of past losses or the ability to determine cause and effect, or causing paranoid or magical thinking that could affect gambling behavior (Grant et al. 2001). For example, there have been anecdotal reports of excessive sweepstakes participation among patients with cognitive dementia (Mendez et al. 2000). Although this is not likely to be an extremely important risk factor in the population, it nevertheless requires further study.

Access to Games of Chance

Adults over age 65 constituted 12.4% of the United States population in the 2000 census (U.S. Census Bureau 2001), and this segment is expected to continue to grow as the population ages and life expectancies increase. As gambling venues multiply, Americans, including older adults, have increasing and more convenient access to various types of gambling. Although rates of gambling are consistently lower among older compared with younger adults (Mok and Hraba 1991; National Opinion Research Center 1999; Pavalko 2002), the increase in access has been reflected in the increase in rates of gambling across all age groups. Surveys taken in the 1970s indicated relatively low gambling participation rates among the elderly; for example, in 1975 only 23% of people over age 65 reported gambling in the previous year, compared with 60%–73% of those in the younger age groups. By 1998, the gap had closed considerably: past-year gambling rates were 50% among those above age 65, compared with 64%–67% among younger age groups (National Opinion Research Center 1999). In addition, the participation in gambling among older Americans will likely continue to increase as younger gamblers age, access to gambling increases, and there is more widespread social acceptance of gambling as a recreational activity.

Patterns of Gambling Behavior

In general, chronological age is negatively associated with gambling prevalence (Mok and Hraba 1991). The limited research on elderly gamblers indicates that people over age 65 differ from younger adults in their reasons for gambling, preferred games, and frequency of gambling.

Reasons for Gambling

Both older and younger adults engage in gambling for a wide variety of reasons. However, research has shown that older adults are generally more likely than younger adults to report gambling to relieve boredom, to be active, or to engage in a social activity (McNeilly and Burke 2000, 2001) and are less likely to report gambling to make money, for the excitement, or for incentives offered by gambling venues (Tarras et al. 2000). Data from the GIBS showed no differences between older and younger gamblers on their motivations for gambling (Desai et al., in press), and at least one marketing study that classified casino gamblers into subtypes based on their motivations found no differences by age (Park et al. 2002). Motivations for gambling, however, may differ substantially across favorite types of gambling, and sample sizes in surveys that covered multiple gambling venues may have been too small to detect such differences. For example, one study comparing community elders with those sampled from casino venues found that casino patrons were less likely to report gambling as a means of socializing with friends (McNeilly and Burke 2000). Another study of nursing home residents, however, found that playing bingo for money was the most common social activity among residents (McNeilly and Burke 2001).

Types of Games Preferred

There is some evidence that there are shifts in the motivations for gambling over age groups and that these shifts may be reflected in preferred games (Mok and Hraba 1991). For example, it has been hypothesized that older adults are attracted to less competitive games such as bingo, lotteries, and slot machines because they are gambling more for the entertainment value than to make money or to beat their opponents. The evidence for this hypothesis is somewhat conflicted and is sparse. One study found that the declining prevalence of gambling behaviors over age groups was much diminished after adjusting for types of gambling (Mok and Hraba 1991). This study also found that elderly respondents were more likely to prefer lotteries and bingo games and to concentrate on a smaller number of games than younger adults. Similarly, surveys of casino patrons have indicated that older adults prefer slot machines to the more competitive card games (Tarras et al. 2000). However, the GIBS found no differences between older and younger respondents on their preferred forms of gambling when grouped by style (e.g., strategic or nonstrategic) or location (e.g., casino or noncasino) (Desai et al., in press). It should be noted that there has been no research on gambling patterns over a lifetime, and the cross-sectional data presented here could be heavily confounded by time-related effects such as selective mortality and the recency of gambling onset. Future research should explore how patterns of gambling change in individuals over a lifetime.

Frequency of Gambling

It has been consistently shown that elderly gamblers differ from younger gamblers in the frequency of play, particularly among those who play bingo and those who travel to casinos. A considerable portion of casino patrons during weekdays and working hours are older, retired adults, and they represent a large portion of casino revenues (Gosker 1999). In addition, elderly adults have been targeted for sweepstakes campaigns (Unger 1999), nursing homes have introduced bingo and other games as a social activity for seniors (McNeilly and Burke 2001), and casinos offer substantial discounts and incentives specifically targeted to seniors (Higgins 2001). The evidence indicates that among seniors who gamble, the frequency of gambling is higher than among younger adult gamblers. For example, data from the GIBS indicated that older gamblers were three times more likely than younger gamblers to gamble daily and were two times more likely to gamble one to three times a week (Desai et al., in press). In a survey of nursing home residents, 23% of residents reported engaging in on-site bingo games more than once a week, and 16% reported taking a day trip to a casino at least once a month (McNeilly and Burke 2001). When comparing elders in gambling venues (casinos and bingo games) with elders in the community, McNeilly and Burke (2000) found that gambling patrons were more likely to report gambling on most types of games at least once a week.

These higher frequencies are likely to be explained by two factors: an increased amount of leisure time available to retirees and the reduction in financial responsibilities (e.g., the support of children) later in life, which may result in relatively higher proportions of disposable income. No matter what the reason, though, such higher frequencies are a potential cause for concern because they may foreshadow higher rates of problem and pathological gambling among seniors.

Health Correlates of Gambling

The impact of gambling, whether recreational or pathological, is also relatively unexamined in the elderly. Early research suggested that gambling increased elders' self-esteem (Campbell 1976) by allowing them to participate more fully in a society that tended to hide them away and exclude them from everyday activities. Recent data from the GIBS found that older gamblers reported better subjective health than their nongambling peers (Desai et al., in press), suggesting that participating in gambling activities may confer some limited health benefits if practiced responsibly. However, these cross-sectional data could be heavily affected by factors such as selection bias, whereby it is not that gambling improves health but that healthier elders are the ones who are more likely to engage in gambling.

Some health effects of gambling may be unique to the elderly, particularly those who engage in casino gambling. First, poor health effects may be associated with sitting for long periods of time, often in smoke-filled environments, eating less frequently than normal, and participating in games that increase heart rates and excitement levels. Although none of these factors would be a particularly immediate concern for younger gamblers, they may be of greater concern for elderly gamblers, who may have diabetes, heart disease, or otherwise poor circulation.

Second, health consequences of large financial losses may be greater among the elderly, who have limited abilities to recoup those losses through work. Large financial losses may be associated with poor medication management due to the inability to purchase medications, loss of independence due to inability to live on diminished means, or increased social isolation resulting from borrowing money or strained family relations resulting from gambling. However, there are no data directly assessing these hypotheses, and further examination is warranted.

Third, elderly women may be at particularly high risk for the development of gambling-related problems and health problems related to gambling. Women make up a majority of the elderly due to their longer life expectancies, and their proportion will likely continue to increase as the population ages. Older women may be at even greater risk for the above-mentioned health effects due to even lower sources of income than older men, a higher likelihood of being widowed and thus socially isolated, and a higher likelihood than elderly men of living with chronic diseases such as diabetes and hypertension. Women of all ages may be more vulnerable than men to the phenomenon of telescoping, whereby they begin gambling later in life but develop gambling-related problems faster than do men (Grant et al. 2001; Potenza et al. 2001; Tavares et al. 2001).

Assessment and Treatment of Pathological Gambling

Elderly patients with problem or pathological gambling may be less likely than younger patients to be identified clinically for several reasons. First, most people with pathological gambling, regardless of age, do not present for treatment, and the elderly may be even less likely to do so. Most studies of problem or pathological gamblers in treatment report mean ages in the mid-40s, suggesting that older gamblers are less likely to seek treatment specifically for gambling.

Instead of seeking specialized treatment, patients with problem and pathological gambling tend to present in primary care settings with more psychosomatic complaints such as back pain, depression, anxiety, or stress-related problems (McCown and Chamberlain 2000; Pavalko 2002; Stewart and Oslin 2001). Among the elderly, who naturally experience more of these physical aches and pains, it may be more difficult to detect an underlying gambling-related problem in a primary care setting (McCown and Chamberlain 2000; Stewart and Oslin 2001). In addition, primary care clinicians are often not very proficient at identifying psychiatric and substance abuse disorders, particularly in the elderly (Stewart and Oslin 2001), and this tendency likely extends to problem and pathological gambling (McCown and Chamberlain 2000).

Third, the elderly may report fewer problems related to gambling, even when asked, for several reasons. Older respondents may attach more of a stigma to disorders such as depression and alcohol dependence and thus may minimize their experience of such symptoms (Sirey et al. 2001a, 2001b). The same may hold true for gambling-related problems such as stress over large losses or family strain due to excessive borrowing. In addition, an exaggerated sense of independence, or the need to retain the limited independence that remains, may prompt greater resistance to recognizing certain symptoms such as financial strain or disruption of family relations (Pavalko 2002). Also, early cognitive decline may interact with the normal course of pathological gambling to create an even more distorted impression of cause and effect: although the majority of pathological gamblers begin to see their gambling as a result, not a cause, of their life difficulties, elderly pathological gamblers may have an even more distorted sense of the causes of their behavior and the effect it has on other people (Pavalko 2002).

No treatments for pathological gambling have been developed specifically for elderly patients. In general, treatment recommendations have involved psychosocial rehabilitation models of treatment, possibly in combination with medications, several of which are being tested for effectiveness. However, some of these recommendations may be particularly challenging to apply to older patients. One recommendation is that patients avoid gambling cues and involvement with other gamblers and that they find suitable leisure activities to substitute for gambling

(Blaszczynski and Silove 1995). This option may be particularly problematic for older adults, who may have developed an elaborate social structure around gambling. Older adults often have fewer social ties (LaVeist et al. 1997; Thompson and Heller 1990), and asking a patient to cut those ties and attempt to replace them could prove to be more challenging in this age group. In addition, if social activities were traditionally heavily related to gambling, finding suitable substitute activities might also be difficult, particularly in the context of limited physical or cognitive capabilities.

A second recommendation is to treat depressive and anxiety symptoms that occur during recovery with appropriate medication (Blaszczynski and Silove 1995). This may also be more challenging in older versus younger adults: older adults may be more resistant to such medications (Chiam 1994), but they also may be taking other medications that would negatively interact with psychotropic medications. A third recommendation is that erroneous beliefs, attitudes, and expectations regarding gambling need to be challenged and corrected (Blaszczynski and Silove 1995). In older patients with diminished cognitive abilities or early symptoms of dementia, Alzheimer's disease, or paranoia, challenging such beliefs might be difficult (Mendez et al. 2000; Unger 1999). Finally, many care providers suggest that attendance at Gamblers Anonymous meetings, whether independent of or in conjunction with other types of treatment, is important, although this view is not necessarily universally endorsed (Blaszczynski and Silove 1995; Pavalko 2002). However, elderly patients with limited capacity for obtaining transportation may experience some difficulty attending such meetings, although better attendance at Gamblers Anonymous has been reported among elderly patients, possibly because of boredom or the availability of more free time (Grant et al. 2001).

Although several pharmacological treatments have shown promise, there are no clearly superior medication treatments for problem and pathological gambling (Grant et al. 2003). Most treatment studies have not separated the effects of treatment by age, and there has been little evidence that treatment effects would differ by age, other factors being equal (e.g., medication interaction effects). However, researchers conducting future treatment studies may want to explore the specific effects over the age span. In addition, some case reports suggest that different sensitivities to pro-dopaminergic drugs might exist, and these might play a role in the treatment of older adults with pathological gambling. Further research could explore the beneficial effect of such drugs specifically for this age group.

Conclusion

Gambling among the elderly has increased dramatically over the past few decades, and older adults represent a major target market for the gambling industry. This combination puts them at potentially increased risk for the development of problem and pathological gambling. Although prevalence rates of gambling-related disorders generally decrease with age, these differences may be diminishing over time. In fact, as gambling becomes more socially acceptable and widely available, rates of problem gambling among the elderly are likely to increase substantially. Older gamblers also have different patterns of gambling than younger adults, and these differences may have implications for the health and well-being of older gamblers. Although the condition is less prevalent than in younger patients, older adults with pathological gambling may have unique treatment challenges as a result of their age, comorbid medical conditions, and attitudes about mental health treatment.

References

American Psychiatric Association: Diagnostic and Statistical Manual of Mental Disorders, 4th Edition. Washington, DC, American Psychiatric Association, 1994

Blaszczynski A, Silove D: Cognitive and behavioral therapies for pathological gambling. J Gambl Stud 11:195–220, 1995

Breen RB, Zimmerman M: Rapid onset of pathological gambling in machine gamblers. J Gambl Stud 18:31–43, 2002

Campbell FF: The future of gambling. The Futurist, April 1, 1976, pp 84–90

Chiam PC: Depression of old age. Singapore Med J 35:404–406, 1994

Custer RL: Profile of the pathological gambler. J Clin Psychiatry 45:35–38, 1984

Desai RA, Maciejewski PK, Dausey DJ, et al: Health correlates of recreational gambling in older adults. Am J Psychiatry (in press)

Gosker E: The marketing of gambling to the elderly. Elder Law Journal 7:184–216, 1999

Grant JE, Kim SW, Brown E: Characteristics of geriatric patients seeking medication treatment for pathologic gambling disorder. J Geriatr Psychiatry Neurol 14:125–129, 2001

Grant JE, Kim SW, Potenza MN: Advances in the pharmacological treatment of pathological gambling. J Gambl Stud 19:85–109, 2003

Gschwandtner U, Aston J, Renaud S, et al: Pathologic gambling in patients with Parkinson's disease. Clin Neuropharmacol 24:170–172, 2001

Higgins J: A comprehensive policy analysis of and recommendations for senior center gambling trips. J Aging Soc Policy 12:73–91, 2001

LaVeist TA, Sellers RM, Brown KA, et al: Extreme social isolation, use of community-based senior support services, and mortality among African American elderly women. Am J Community Psychol 25:721–732, 1997

McCown WG, Chamberlain LL: Best Possible Odds: Contemporary Treatment Strategies for Gambling Disorders. New York, Wiley, 2000

McNeilly DP, Burke WJ: Late life gambling: the attitudes and behaviors of older adults. J Gambl Stud 16:393–415, 2000

McNeilly DP, Burke WJ: Gambling as a social activity of older adults. Int J Aging Hum Dev 52:19–28, 2001

McNeilly DP, Burke WJ: Disposable time and disposable income: problem casino gambling behavior in older adults. Journal of Clinical Geropsychology 8:75–85, 2002

Mendez MF, Bronstein YL, Christine DL: Excessive sweepstakes participation by persons with dementia. J Am Geriatr Soc 48:855–856, 2000

Mok WP, Hraba J: Age and gambling behavior: a declining and shifting pattern of participation. J Gambl Stud 7:313–335, 1991

Molina JA, Sainz-Artiga MJ, Fraile A, et al: Pathologic gambling in Parkinson's disease: a behavioral manifestation of pharmacologic treatment? Mov Disord 15:869–872, 2000

National Opinion Research Center: Gambling Impact and Behavior Study: Report to the National Gambling Impact Study Commission. Chicago, IL, National Opinion Research Center at the University of Chicago, 1999. Available at: http://www.norc.uchicago.edu/new/gamb-fin.htm. Accessed December 13, 2003.

Park M, Yang X, Lee B, et al: Segmenting casino gamblers by involvement profiles: a Colorado example. Tourism Management 23:55–65, 2002

Pavalko RM: Problem gambling among older people, in Treating Alcohol and Drug Abuse in the Elderly. Edited by Gurnack AM, Atkinson RM, Osgood NJ. New York, Springer, 2002, pp 190–213

Potenza MN, Steinberg MA, McLaughlin SD, et al: Gender-related differences in the characteristics of problem gamblers using a gambling helpline. Am J Psychiatry 158:1500–1505, 2001

Seedat S, Kesler S, Niehaus DJH, et al: Pathological gambling behaviour: emergence secondary to treatment of Parkinson's disease with dopaminergic agents. Depress Anxiety 11:185–186, 2000

Sirey JA, Bruce ML, Alexopoulos GS, et al: Perceived stigma as a predictor of treatment discontinuation in young and older outpatients with depression. Am J Psychiatry 158:479–481, 2001a

Sirey JA, Bruce ML, Alexopoulos GS, et al: Stigma as a barrier to recovery: perceived stigma and patient-rated severity of illness as predictors of antidepressant drug adherence. Psychiatr Serv 52:1615–1620, 2001b

Stewart D, Oslin DW: Recognition and treatment of late-life addictions in medical settings. Journal of Clinical Geropsychology 7:145–158, 2001

Tarras J, Singh AJ, Moufakkir O: The profile and motivations of elderly women gamblers. Gaming Research and Review Journal 5:33–46, 2000

Tavares H, Zilberman ML, Beites FJ, et al: Gender differences in gambling progression. J Gambl Stud 17:151–159, 2001

Thompson MG, Heller K: Facets of support related to well-being: quantitative social isolation and perceived family support in a sample of elderly women. Psychol Aging 5:535–544, 1990

Unger BL: Deceptive Mail: Consumers' Problems Appear Substantial. Washington, DC, U.S. General Accounting Office, 1999, pp 1–22

U.S. Census Bureau: Resident Population Estimates of the United States by Age and Sex: April 1, 1990 to July 1, 1999, With Short-Term Projection to November 1, 2000. Washington, DC, U.S. Census Bureau, 2001. Available at: http://eire.census.gov/popest/archives/national/nation2/intfile2-1.txt. Accessed December 13, 2003.

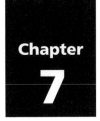

Chapter

7

Gender Differences

Jon E. Grant, J.D., M.D., M.P.H.
Suck Won Kim, M.D.

The notion of meaningful differences between men and women in various aspects of pathological gambling is a topic that has received increasing attention over the past 5 years. Although pathological gambling is considered to be primarily a male problem, the recent focus on pathological gambling in women has brought attention to important gender differences in epidemiology, phenomenology, psychiatric comorbidity, and biology. These differences have important treatment implications. In this chapter, findings concerning gender differences are reviewed within a clinical context.

Case 1

Michael, a 29-year-old man, started gambling with his father at age 15. Michael's father introduced him to poker and encouraged him to bet on sporting events. Michael gradually began playing poker with friends for money. Although he would occasionally not have money for extracurricular activities because of his gambling, his gambling did not cause significant problems for him until he was about 24 years old. At that time, Michael began going to casinos. Michael reported that his urges to gamble were often triggered by advertisements for the local casino and by fantasies of winning large amounts of money.

Even with a time-intensive career in accounting, Michael played blackjack approximately three evenings each week. Always intending on staying only 2 or 3 hours at the casino, Michael would most often play blackjack for 8–10 hours each evening. In addition, he began gambling with larger amounts of money. His work suffered as a result of his gambling. He would be too tired from staying at the casino late or too preoccupied with almost constant thoughts of winning back his lost money, that his decreased attention to work detail was noticeable to coworkers and his employer.

His family life also suffered. Although he promised himself and his wife that he would remember and be available for family events, Michael usually chose gambling over these family activities. Michael would then lie to his wife about his whereabouts. The deception led to guilt and marital strain. With fear of impending divorce and unemployment, Michael sought help for gambling.

Case 2

Susan did not start gambling until she was 48 years old. Susan remembers the first time she went to a casino. Friends asked her to join them for dinner and entertainment. Susan and her friends began to go to the casino twice a month. Susan began playing nickel slot machines. Because winning at the nickel machines gradually lost its excitement, over the next 2 years Susan found that only dollar slot machines produced a "thrill."

Within 2 years of starting casino gambling, Susan felt she had a problem. Susan no longer wanted to go to the casino with her friends. She found them too distracting and reported that they did not take gambling seriously. Instead, Susan started going by herself. This also allowed Susan to go to the casino more frequently and to stay for longer periods of time.

Susan reported that her interest in gambling would often be prompted by her mood. If she was feeling anxious due to work or feeling sad or lonely because of problems within her marriage, Susan would choose to go to the casino. In fact, when stress at work was at its highest, Susan would often choose to leave work early. Because of her frequent absences, Susan eventually lost her job. Because she avoided telling her husband about her problem until it got out of hand, Susan's marriage eventually ended in divorce.

When her mood was good and her anxiety minimal, however, Susan could go for weeks without gambling. At these times, Susan felt that she had control over her problem and that treatment was unnecessary. Untreated, the behavior would come back as quickly as it had left. Reluctantly, Susan sought treatment after a friend pressured her to do so.

Epidemiology

Community Populations

A recent meta-analysis of the available literature concluded that 2.2 million adults (1.6%) in North America have pathological gambling, with an additional 5.3 million adults (3.9%) being at risk for developing the disorder (Shaffer et al. 1999). In epidemiological studies, women represent approximately 32% of the pathological gamblers in the United States (Cunningham-Williams et al. 1998; National Gambling Impact Study Commission 1999; Shaffer et al. 1999; Volberg 1994).

Do these epidemiological findings accurately reflect the extent of pathological gambling among women? The prevalence rates may instead be associated with the social norms that influence gambling behavior. Before the increased accessibility of casinos and lotteries, gambling options involved mainly the male-dominated spheres of sports, cards, and racing (Ladd and Petry 2002). Therefore, women were arguably less likely to develop gambling problems than they might be today, and a cohort phenomenon may be reflected in the findings of epidemiological studies. As younger females are exposed to more available forms of gambling, the percentage of females with pathological gambling may approach or equal that of males.

Clinical Populations

The gender ratio in clinical populations suggests a higher percentage of women seeking treatment for pathological gambling than has been found in community samples. Seven double-blind studies (Blanco et al. 2002; Grant et al. 2003; Haller and Hinterhuber 1994; Hollander et al. 1992, 2000; Kim et al. 2001, 2002), five open-label or single-blind studies (Hollander et al. 1998; Kim and Grant 2001a; Pallanti et al. 2002a, 2002b; Zimmerman et al. 2002), and two case reports (Crockford and el-Guebaly 1998; Moskowitz 1980) of pharmacological interventions have been published. These studies enrolled a total of 308 subjects, of whom 129 (41.9%) were female—a higher percentage of females than has been found in epidemiological studies. These findings are similar to those for other mental disorders and reflect an apparent tendency for women compared with men to be more likely to seek mental health treatment.

The higher percentage of females found in the treatment studies still may not adequately reflect the extent of gambling problems among women. Although reasons have not been rigorously examined, there has long been a suggestion that women are underrepresented in treatment programs (Mark and Lesieur 1992). In part, this finding may reflect female pathological gamblers' decreased willingness to seek treatment for gambling problems (Grant and Kim 2002; Ladd and Petry 2002). Alcohol treatment literature suggests that women have gender-specific barriers to treatment such as lack of funding, child care and custody issues, and difficulty obtaining transportation (Brady and Randall 1999). Whether similar barriers exist for female pathological gamblers seeking treatment is currently unknown. Another explanation drawn from the alcohol treatment literature is that women may seek treatment after a severe episode of gambling, whereas men seek treatment after a more chronic period (Ladd and Petry 2002). Whether some women have not sought treatment because they simply have not yet "hit bottom" is unclear, but this difference in motivation for treatment may offer clues to the gender ratios found in clinical samples.

The gender ratio of subjects in clinical samples, however, may be influenced by age. The age of the clinical populations in the pharmacological studies may have skewed the numbers closer to an equal gender ratio. The approximate mean age of the subjects in these studies was 40–45 years. Two studies of older pathological gamblers have found that a high percentage of women in these older-age cohorts seeks treatment (Grant et al. 2001; Petry et al. 2002). As the case examples at the beginning of the chapter demonstrate, women tend to start gambling at a later age, and so the age of the sample may influence the gender ratio. Thus in clinical settings, women, particularly of middle to older age, should be screened for pathological gambling because it may be more common than was previously estimated.

Phenomenology

Course of Illness

The case examples presented above reflect many of the characteristic differences between male and female pathological gamblers. Perhaps the most replicated finding in studies has been that the course of illness seems to be different for women. The interval between the age of initially gambling for money and the age of recognizing problems due to gambling seems to be shorter for women (Grant and Kim 2002; Ibáñez et al. 2003; Ladd and Petry 2002; Martins et al. 2002; Potenza et al. 2001; Tavares et al. 2001). This accelerated development of addiction in women, the so-called telescoping effect, has been documented in other addictive disorders such as alcohol use disorders and opiate dependence (Brady and Randall 1999; Randall et al. 1999).

Triggers to Gambling

Female pathological gamblers are also more likely to report that they gamble as a means of escaping from stressful or unsatisfying life situations or from states of depression, whereas men often report urges to gamble unrelated to their emotional state (Grant and Kim 2002; Ladd and Petry

2002; Potenza et al. 2001; Trevorrow and Moore 1998). Although some studies have found that female pathological gamblers have high rates of mood disorders that might explain the triggers for gambling (Ibáñez et al. 2003), similar rates of mood disorders have been found among samples of predominantly male pathological gamblers (Black and Moyer 1998). Social situations may also explain why affective state is a more prominent trigger for women. Ladd and Petry (2002) suggested that the home environment may be more unstable, stressful, and unsupportive for female pathological gamblers.

The emotional state that female pathological gamblers report as the trigger to gambling appears to correlate with the type of gambling women prefer. Although choice of gambling activity depends on availability, women tend to prefer and to develop problems with nonstrategic forms of gambling such as bingo or slot machines (Grant and Kim 2002; Potenza et al. 2001; Tavares et al. 2001). Nonstrategic forms of gambling may be more escape oriented, whereas a man's choice of strategic gambling may be more action oriented (for example, sports gambling or blackjack) (Potenza et al. 2001). Furthermore, the action-oriented gambling may also reflect a higher level of sensation seeking among male pathological gamblers (Blaszczynski et al. 1997; Vitaro et al. 1997).

Although women often report pronounced mood symptoms as the prompt for their gambling behavior, many will not meet diagnostic criteria for a mood disorder. These women, however, may have subclinical mood symptoms that predispose them to gambling. Therefore, it is clinically important to inquire not only about possible depression and anxiety but also about the emotional context in which the woman finds herself when gambling. The alcohol treatment literature advises that women may require more assistance in finding alternatives to drinking to cope with negative affect (Rubin et al. 1996). Having patients maintain a diary of their mood and gambling behavior may be helpful in demonstrating a possible link between these factors and identifying high-risk times for gambling. If the emotional cues for gambling are not identified, treatment may not focus on the cause of the disordered gambling.

Comorbidity

Studies have consistently reported that subjects with pathological gambling experience high rates of lifetime mood (60%–76%) (Linden et al. 1986; McCormick et al. 1984; Roy et al. 1988), anxiety (16%–40%) (Crockford and el-Guebaly 1998; Ibáñez et al. 2001), and substance use (33%–63%) disorders (Black and Moyer 1998; Grant et al. 2002). In terms of gender differences in comorbidity, one study found that male pathological gamblers were more likely to have a current alcohol use disorder, whereas females were more likely to have a comorbid mood disorder (Ibáñez et al. 2001). The higher rates of comorbid mood disorders among female pathological gamblers may also explain the higher reported rates of attempted suicide among women with these disorders (Potenza et al. 2001). Potenza et al. (2001) also found that male gamblers were more likely to report problems with drug use. Consistent with these findings, Ladd and Petry (2002) found that male pathological gamblers were more likely to have had prior treatment for substance abuse than were female gamblers.

Other aspects of comorbidity have been found less consistently in the literature. For example, one study found that female gamblers were more likely to report anxiety due to their gambling (Potenza et al. 2001). Differences in scores on the Hamilton Anxiety Scale, however, have not been found to differ between genders (Grant et al. 2003). Also, there is no evidence that female compared with male pathological gamblers experience higher rates of categorical anxiety disorders (Ibáñez et al. 2003). Rates of personality disorders also do not differ between genders, although there is some indication that antisocial traits may be higher among male pathological gamblers (Ibáñez et al. 2003).

In critically reviewing the area of gender differences in comorbidity with pathological gambling, physicians must keep in mind the gender differences in psychiatric disorders in the general population. Epidemiological surveys indicate that in the general population, affective disorders are more common in women (Kessler et al. 1994), whereas alcohol use disorders are more common in men (Helzer et al. 1991). Thus, it is possible that the gender differences in comorbidity in pathological gamblers reflect the gender differences for these psychiatric disorders found in the general population.

Problems Due to Gambling

Problems arising from gambling behavior may differ based on gender. Although legal problems tend to be fairly common in patients with pathological gambling (Grant and Kim 2001), recent studies have examined illegal behavior in gambling subjects and have reported inconsistent findings. For example, one study determined that male pathological gamblers reported more illegal activities (Ladd and Petry 2002). A separate study, however, found similar rates of acknowledgment of gambling-related illegal activities reported by male and female problem gamblers (21.4% of women and 22.3% of men) (Potenza et al. 2000). Two other studies also found no differences in illegal behavior based on gender

(Grant and Kim 2001; Ibáñez et al. 2003). Finally, two studies have found that male gamblers are more likely to report illegal behaviors resulting in arrest than are female gamblers (Ladd and Petry 2002; Potenza et al. 2001).

Although some studies have found that female problem gamblers are more likely to have financial problems due to gambling (Potenza et al. 2001), high rates of financial problems have been found in both groups (Grant and Kim 2001; Ibáñez et al. 2003; Potenza et al. 2001). In particular, the majority of both male and female pathological gamblers report credit card problems secondary to gambling (Grant and Kim 2001; Potenza et al. 2001), and approximately one-fourth of both groups have filed for bankruptcy due to gambling debt (Grant and Kim 2001). In addition, Ibáñez et al. (2003) found that men were more likely to have marital consequences from their gambling than were women.

Personality Differences

Although the number of categorical personality disorders does not appear to differ between male and female pathological gamblers (Ibáñez et al. 2003), gender may still influence personality characteristics of pathological gamblers. The extent to which male and female gamblers differ with respect to personality traits, however, remains unclear. One study found that pathological gamblers reported significantly greater novelty seeking and impulsiveness than control subjects without pathological gambling, and these traits did not distinguish male and female pathological gamblers (Kim and Grant 2001b). Another study, using a different scale to assess personality traits, found that male compared with female pathological gamblers were more sensation seeking and more likely to experiment (Ibáñez et al. 2003). With only two studies having been conducted using different scales, meaningful comments concerning personality differences in male and female pathological gamblers require data from further investigations.

Patterns of Heredity

Behavioral genetic studies can provide estimates of the extent of genetic versus environmental contributions to specific behaviors and conditions by contrasting the concordance of these behaviors and conditions between monozygotic and dizygotic twin pairs. In one study of male twins, familial factors (both genetic and environmental) explained 56%–62% of the occurrence of pathological gambling. The lifetime prevalence rates of pathological gambling were 22.6% for monozygotic twins and 9.8% for dizygotic twins (Eisen et al. 1998).

A second twin study, again using only male pathological gamblers, specifically examined the association between pathological gambling and alcohol use disorders (Slutske et al. 2000). In that study, 12%–20% of the genetic variation in risk for pathological gambling was held in common by both pathological gambling and alcohol use disorders. In addition, genetic factors accounted for 64% of the overlap between these two disorders. The study also found that 3%–8% of the nonshared environmental variation was common for both conditions. In the same cohort, it was also found that the co-occurrence of pathological gambling and antisocial behavior disorders was greater than that due to chance and that the co-occurrence was at least partially due to a common genetic vulnerability (Slutske et al. 2001).

Because these studies involved only male pathological gamblers, it remains unclear how these findings may apply to female pathological gamblers. However, one study produced a hint about differences in genetic influences with the finding that rates of first-degree relatives with alcohol use disorders were equally high among both male and female probands with pathological gambling (Grant and Kim 2001).

Other genetic differences have also been examined. One study found a possible significant association between pathological gambling in females and the dopamine D_4 receptor gene *(DRD4)* that leads to less efficient functioning of this particular dopamine receptor (Perez de Castro et al. 1997). In addition, serotonergic functioning has been implicated in pathological gambling, and a possible association has been discovered between DNA polymorphisms in monoamine oxidase A genes and a subgroup of males with severe pathological gambling (Ibáñez et al. 2000). Another finding related to serotonergic function is that male pathological gamblers may more frequently have a less functional variant of a polymorphism of the serotonin transporter gene (Perez de Castro et al. 1999). These findings suggest a contribution of genetic factors in the pathophysiology of pathological gambling and suggest that these genetic factors may differ based on gender. Further studies are needed of the genetic differences between female and male pathological gamblers.

Access and Responsiveness to Treatment

Little systematic research on gender-specific treatment response has been conducted. Assuming that both male and female pathological gamblers seek treatment, however, there appears to be little difference in their responses to treatment. Only 4 of the 12 pharmacotherapy studies cited above (see "Clinical Populations") included analysis of response based on gender. Trials of the antidepressants nefazodone and paroxetine and of the opioid antagonist naltrexone did not result in any gender differences in response to medication (Grant et al. 2003; Kim et al. 2001, 2002; Pallanti et al. 2002a). In only one trial (involving the selective serotonin reuptake inhibitor fluvoxamine) was it found that males had a significantly better response to treatment than those receiving placebo (Blanco et al. 2002). Of the two studies of cognitive-behavioral therapy, neither assessed response with respect to gender (Ladouceur et al. 2001; Sylvain et al. 1997). In the reports published to date, the relatively small samples studied have provided limited power to detect gender-related differences in treatment response. It is anticipated that future studies involving larger samples will provide additional insight into optimal treatments for men and women with pathological gambling.

Treatment Implications

A better understanding of gender differences in treatment response may help in the development of more efficient strategies for prevention and treatment. For example, because females progress to pathological gambling at a faster rate than males, treatment should arguably be initiated earlier in females, ideally at the first indication of gambling addiction. Gender differences in triggers to gambling have treatment implications. An appropriate treatment for women should target affective symptoms (including those that do not meet criteria for an Axis I mood disorder) and should address troubling aspects of the home environment. Conversely, the best treatment for men may be to tailor cognitive-behavioral therapy to a variety of sensation-seeking behaviors. Also, comorbidity of alcohol use disorders in male pathological gamblers may require more intense treatment, because these patients are likely to have more functional impairment and a poorer prognosis than those with either condition alone (Bukstein et al. 1989).

Conclusion

Based on the recent research, a greater appreciation for the differences between male and female pathological gamblers is emerging. Women tend to start gambling later in life but appear to develop pathological gambling at a faster rate after starting to gamble. Women may use gambling to self-medicate mood disturbances, whereas for men a greater component of sensation seeking or competitive risk taking may predominate. Men are more likely to have comorbid alcohol use disorders. Overall, women and men appear to respond equally well to both pharmacotherapy and psychotherapy, although relatively few large treatment studies of pathological gambling have been performed that would permit direct examination of gender-related differences.

Gender differences have significant treatment implications. The telescoping effect for females suggests a need for early intervention after the onset of gambling and a greater index of suspicion for the presence of gambling problems in women in middle and older age groups. Similarly, data suggest that prevention and treatment efforts should be tailored for younger age groups, which have disproportionately high numbers of male problem and pathological gamblers. Gender-related barriers to treatment should be addressed across age groups to encourage more pathological gamblers to seek, enter into, and benefit from treatment. Comorbidity, particularly alcohol use disorders in male pathological gamblers, may require more intense interventions. The comparison of male and female pathological gamblers promises to be a fruitful one to improve treatment outcomes for both genders.

References

Black DW, Moyer T: Clinical features and psychiatric comorbidity of subjects with pathological gambling behavior. Psychiatr Serv 49:1434–1439, 1998

Blanco C, Petkova E, Ibáñez A, et al: A pilot placebo-controlled study of fluvoxamine for pathological gambling. Ann Clin Psychiatry 14:9–15, 2002

Blaszczynski A, Steel Z, McConaghy N: Impulsivity in pathological gambling: the antisocial impulsivist. Addiction 92:75–87, 1997

Brady KT, Randall CL: Gender differences in substance use disorders. Psychiatr Clin North Am 22:241–252, 1999

Bukstein OG, Brent DA, Kaminer Y: Comorbidity of substance abuse and other psychiatric disorders in adolescents. Am J Psychiatry 146:1131–1141, 1989

Crockford DN, el-Guebaly N: Psychiatric comorbidity in pathological gambling: a critical review. Can J Psychiatry 43:43–50, 1998

Cunningham-Williams RM, Cottler LB, Compton WM III, et al: Taking chances: problem gamblers and mental health disorders—results from the St. Louis Epidemiologic Catchment Area Study. Am J Public Health 88:1093–1096, 1998

Eisen SA, Lin N, Lyons MJ, et al: Familial influences on gambling behavior: an analysis of 3359 twin pairs. Addiction 93:1375–1384, 1998

Grant JE, Kim SW: Demographic and clinical features of 131 adult pathological gamblers. J Clin Psychiatry 62:957–962, 2001

Grant JE, Kim SW: Gender differences in pathological gamblers seeking medication treatment. Compr Psychiatry 43:56–62, 2002

Grant JE, Kim SW, Brown E: Characteristics of geriatric patients seeking medication treatment for pathologic gambling disorder. J Geriatr Psychiatry Neurol 14:125–129, 2001

Grant JE, Kushner MG, Kim SW: Pathological gambling and alcohol use disorder. Alcohol Res Health 26:143–150, 2002

Grant JE, Kim SW, Potenza MN, et al: Paroxetine treatment of pathological gambling: a multi-center randomized controlled trial. Int Clin Psychopharmacol 18:243–249, 2003

Haller R, Hinterhuber H: Treatment of pathological gambling with carbamazepine (letter). Pharmacopsychiatry 27:129, 1994

Helzer JE, Burnam A, McEvoy LT: Alcohol abuse and dependence, in Psychiatric Disorders in America: The Epidemiologic Catchment Area Study. Edited by Robins LN, Regier DA. New York, Free Press, 1991, pp 81–115

Hollander E, Frenkel M, DeCaria C, et al: Treatment of pathological gambling with clomipramine (letter). Am J Psychiatry 149:710–711, 1992

Hollander E, DeCaria CM, Mari E, et al: Short-term, single-blind fluvoxamine treatment of pathological gambling. Am J Psychiatry 155:1781–1783, 1998

Hollander E, DeCaria CM, Finkell JN, et al: A randomized double-blind fluvoxamine/placebo crossover trial in pathologic gambling. Biol Psychiatry 47:813–817, 2000

Ibáñez A, de Castro IP, Fernandez-Piqueras J, et al: Pathological gambling and DNA polymorphic markers at MAO-A and MAO-B genes. Mol Psychiatry 5:105–109, 2000

Ibáñez A, Blanco C, Donahue E, et al: Psychiatric comorbidity in pathological gamblers seeking treatment. Am J Psychiatry 158:1733–1735, 2001

Ibáñez A, Blanco C, Moreyra P, et al: Gender differences in pathological gambling. J Clin Psychiatry 64:295–301, 2003

Kessler RC, McGonagle KA, Zhao S, et al: Lifetime and 12-month prevalence of DSM-III-R psychiatric disorders in the United States: results from the National Comorbidity Survey. Arch Gen Psychiatry 51:8–19, 1994

Kim SW, Grant JE: An open naltrexone treatment study of pathological gambling disorder. Int Clin Psychopharmacol 16:285–289, 2001a

Kim SW, Grant JE: Personality dimensions in pathological gambling disorder and obsessive-compulsive disorder. Psychiatry Res 104:205–212, 2001b

Kim SW, Grant JE, Adson DE, et al: Double-blind naltrexone and placebo comparison study in the treatment of pathological gambling. Biol Psychiatry 49:914–921, 2001

Kim SW, Grant JE, Adson DE, et al: A double-blind, placebo-controlled study of the efficacy and safety of paroxetine in the treatment of pathological gambling disorder. J Clin Psychiatry 63:501–507, 2002

Ladd GT, Petry NM: Gender differences among pathological gamblers seeking treatment. Exp Clin Psychopharmacol 10:302–309, 2002

Ladouceur R, Sylvain C, Boutin C, et al: Cognitive treatment of pathological gambling. J Nerv Ment Dis 189:774–780, 2001

Linden RD, Pope HG Jr, Jonas JM: Pathological gambling and major affective disorder: preliminary findings. J Clin Psychiatry 47:201–203, 1986

Mark ME, Lesieur HR: A feminist critique of problem gambling research. Br J Addiction 87:549–565, 1992

Martins SS, Lobo DS, Tavares H, et al: Pathological gambling in women: a review. Rev Hosp Clin Fac Med Sao Paulo 57:235–242, 2002

McCormick RA, Russo AM, Ramirez LF, et al: Affective disorders among pathological gamblers seeking treatment. Am J Psychiatry 141:215–218, 1984

Moskowitz JA: Lithium and lady luck: use of lithium carbonate in compulsive gambling. NY State J Med 80:785–788, 1980

National Gambling Impact Study Commission: National Gambling Impact Study Commission Final Report. Washington, DC, National Gambling Impact Study Commission, 1999. Available at: http://govinfo.library.unt.edu/ngisc/reports/fullrpt.html. Accessed December 14, 2003.

Pallanti S, Baldini Rossi N, Sood E, et al: Nefazodone treatment of pathological gambling: a prospective open-label controlled trial. J Clin Psychiatry 63:1034–1039, 2002a

Pallanti S, Quercioli L, Sood E, et al: Lithium and valproate treatment of pathological gambling: a randomized single-blind study. J Clin Psychiatry 63:559–564, 2002b

Perez de Castro I, Ibáñez A, Torres P, et al: Genetic association study between pathological gambling and a functional DNA polymorphism at the D4 receptor gene. Pharmacogenetics 7:345–348, 1997

Perez de Castro I, Ibáñez A, Saiz-Ruiz J, et al: Genetic contribution to pathological gambling: possible association between a functional DNA polymorphism at the serotonin transporter gene (5-HTT) and affected men. Pharmacogenetics 9:397–400, 1999

Petry NM: A comparison of young, middle-aged, and older adult treatment-seeking gamblers. The Gerontologist 42:92–99, 2002

Potenza MN, Steinberg MA, McLaughlin SD, et al: Illegal behaviors in problem gambling: analysis of data from a gambling helpline. J Am Acad Psychiatry Law 28:389–403, 2000

Potenza MN, Steinberg MA, McLaughlin SD, et al: Gender-related differences in the characteristics of problem gamblers using a gambling helpline. Am J Psychiatry 158:1500–1505, 2001

Randall CL, Roberts JS, Del Boca FK, et al: Telescoping of landmark events associated with drinking: a gender comparison. J Stud Alcohol 60:252–260, 1999

Roy A, Adinoff B, Roehrich L, et al: Pathological gambling: a psychobiological study. Arch Gen Psychiatry 45:369–373, 1988

Rubin A, Stout RL, Longabaugh R: Gender differences in relapse situations. Addiction 91 (suppl):111–120, 1996

Shaffer HJ, Hall MN, Vander Bilt J: Estimating the prevalence of disordered gambling behavior in the United States and Canada: a research synthesis. Am J Public Health 89:1369–1376, 1999

Slutske WS, Eisen S, True WR, et al: Common genetic vulnerability for pathological gambling and alcohol dependence in men. Arch Gen Psychiatry 57:666–673, 2000

Slutske WS, Eisen S, Xian H, et al: A twin study of the association between pathological gambling and antisocial personality disorder. J Abnorm Psychol 110:297–308, 2001

Sylvain C, Ladouceur R, Boisvert JM: Cognitive and behavioral treatment of pathological gambling: a controlled study. J Consult Clin Psychol 65:727–732, 1997

Tavares H, Zilberman ML, Beites FJ, et al: Gender differences in gambling progression. J Gambl Stud 17:151–159, 2001

Trevorrow K, Moore S: The association between loneliness, social isolation, and women's electronic gaming machine gambling. J Gambl Stud 14:263–284, 1998

Vitaro F, Arseneault L, Trenblay RE: Dispositional predictors of problem gambling in male adolescents. Am J Psychiatry 154:1769–1770, 1997

Volberg RA: The prevalence and demographics of pathological gamblers: implications for public health. Am J Public Health 84:237–241, 1994

Zimmerman M, Breen RB, Posternak MA: An open-label study of citalopram in the treatment of pathological gambling. J Clin Psychiatry 63:44–48, 2002

Part

III

Etiology

Behavioral Understanding

Kenneth Abrams, Ph.D.
Matt G. Kushner, Ph.D.

In this chapter we explore behavioral, cognitive, and dispositional theories of the etiology of pathological gambling. Behavioral and social-learning theorists have focused on the role of direct and vicarious reinforcement in the development and maintenance of gambling behaviors. Cognitive theorists have focused on information processing biases that inflate subjective estimates of winning or that otherwise promote the persistence of gambling. Dispositional traits such as impulsiveness, sensation seeking, neuroticism, and extraversion as well as antisocial personality traits have also been postulated as being significant in the development of pathological gambling. After reviewing literature relevant to each of these perspectives, we conclude by considering the associations of the psychological models with neurobiological systems that have been linked to pathological gambling.

Operant Conditioning

Positive-Reinforcement Models

Positive reinforcement refers to the introduction of a hedonically positive consequence that strengthens a preceding response. From an operant standpoint, the variable ratio of wins and losses built into institutional gambling provides a particularly pathogenic formulation. The quintessential positive reinforcer of gambling behavior is winning money. The intermittent reinforcement (i.e., winning money on an unpredictably variable ratio) of gambling behavior describes a schedule of reinforcement that is particularly resistant to extinction, even in the absence of reinforcement over many trials. Furthermore, McCown and Chamberlain (2000) observed that extinction may be an especially slow process with gambling because both the frequency and magnitude of reinforcement may vary over time.

In addition to money, theorists have posited a range of reinforcers available to gamblers that may serve to initiate and perpetuate the behavior (e.g., Hayano 1982; Ocean and Smith 1993). These include social reinforcers (e.g., interaction with employees and other players), material reinforcers (e.g., drinks and other goods and services provided for players), ambient reinforcers (e.g., the wide array of visual and auditory stimuli present in many casinos), cognitive reinforcers (e.g., "near misses" such as being one card away from a large payout), and even physiological arousal.

Another idea related to operant conditioning involves the importance of big wins (typically defined as either exceeding one's annual salary or grossly exceeding one's expectations) early in one's gambling career. Two retrospective studies have found that a disproportionate number of pathological gamblers report experiencing big wins early in their gambling careers (Snyder 1978; Walker 1992). Another study showed that among individuals who gambled and experienced the same overall number of wins, those who experienced them sooner viewed themselves as more successful and played for longer periods of time (Coventry and Norman 1997).

Negative-Reinforcement Models

One theory based on *negative reinforcement* (i.e., involving the removal of a punishing stimulus) hypothesizes that initiating but not completing a habitual behavior leads to uncomfortable states of arousal (McConaghy 1980). Applied to gambling, this would imply that a frequent player who has begun playing but has not yet accrued significant winnings (i.e., "completed" the behavior) might continue placing bets to experience relief from aversive arousal. It should be noted that this theory has features in common with drive-reduction theory and could explain why gambling behavior continues within a gambling session despite continuous losses.

In another negative reinforcement–based model, Jacobs (1986) argues that addictions in general (and gambling in particular) may allow individuals who are chronically either overaroused or underaroused to achieve an optimal arousal level. In one test of this theory, researchers assessed personality traits, arousal patterns, and motivations to gamble in 12 problem machine gamblers and 13 problem horse-racing gamblers (Cocco et al. 1995). The researchers found that horse-race gamblers scored higher than poker machine gamblers on boredom proneness and sensation seeking and preferred increased arousal levels. The researchers concluded that these gamblers selected horse racing as a gambling venue because some degree of skill is involved and that they placed bets to increase their excitement and arousal levels to more desired levels.

The machine gamblers in the aforementioned study were more anxious as a group and preferred lower arousal levels. By narrowing their attention, gambling may provide these individuals with an opportunity to distract themselves from an array of life problems and thereby to escape uncomfortably high arousal levels (Lopez Viets and Miller 1997). These gamblers may have been able to reattribute residual elevated arousal levels as stemming from "playing a game" (a low-stress attribution) versus "attempting to win money" (a high-stress attribution), further serving to negatively reinforce (i.e., through relief) their gambling behavior.

A final negative-reinforcement model is based on the "self-medication" model. A number of studies have found elevated rates of depression and anxiety disorders in pathological gamblers (e.g., Blaszczynski and McConaghy 1989). The lifetime prevalence rate for mood disorders in pathological gamblers may be as high as 60%, and the rate for anxiety disorders may be as high as 40% (Black and Moyer 1998). Depressed or anxious individuals may gamble to distract themselves from life stressors and unpleasant cognitions. Persons who are depressed or anxious may also view gambling winnings as a means of significant symptom relief and gambling losses as a relatively minor setback (Sharpe 2002). Ironically, problems resulting directly from gambling (e.g., financial distress, relationship problems, criminal activity) may in turn lead to even more gambling in a misguided attempt at symptom management (Sharpe 2002).

Vicarious Learning

Social learning theory asserts that individuals have a propensity to imitate behaviors they observe that are followed by reinforcement. Thus, individuals who observe the gambling behavior of friends, family members, or even role models on television may be more likely to gamble themselves. Big lottery winners are much more likely to receive media attention than are the millions of lottery losers. The potential for media-based vicarious reinforcement of gambling behavior is greater than that for media-based vicarious punishment. Also, hearing of big wins made by others (e.g., lottery winners or big casino winners) is especially salient, relative to hearing about people losing. In short, whereas losing tends to be a private affair, the public is bombarded with images of big winners that can serve as potent vicarious sources of positive reinforcement of gambling behavior.

Cognitive Factors

Several researchers have outlined theories of the etiology of pathological gambling by linking thinking errors (or cognitive distortions) directly to pathological gambling behavior (e.g., Rogers 1998; Toneatto 1999). This effort has identified a substantial list of specific thinking errors that are believed to worsen, if not directly cause, problem gambling: 1) superstitious beliefs (e.g., believing in good-luck objects or behaviors); 2) interpretive biases (e.g., attributing wins to skill and losses to flukes; wrongly believing that a series of losses increases the chance of a subsequent win); 3) temporal telescoping (e.g., expecting that naturally occurring—that is, probabilistically expected—wins will happen sooner rather than later and for oneself rather than for others); 4) selective memory (e.g., remembering wins while ignoring losses, or totaling wins without correcting for amounts lost); and 5) illusory correlations (i.e., ascribing causal force to contextual stimuli that are only incidentally associated with a win or loss).

Many gamblers have an affinity for long-shot bets, even when the expected payoff from such bets is extremely low. Daniel Kahneman and Vernon Smith (co-winners of the 2002 Nobel Prize in economics) argued that people make different decisions depending on how a risk is conceptualized (Tversky and Kahneman 1981; McCabe and Smith 2000). In their view, people will avoid risks to ensure gains (even small gains) but will take risks (even big risks) to avoid definite losses. This model predicts that those focused on avoiding definite loss (e.g., "you can't win if you don't play") may be willing to make seemingly illogical bets.

The *sunk-cost effect* has been defined as an increased willingness to engage in behavior one ordinarily might not engage in because of money or time already invested in the process (Arkes and Ayton 1999). For example, pathological gamblers who lose large sums of money at the front end of a gambling session may imagine that the entire net loss could be recouped with a single large payout. Therefore, gambling behavior may continue because of time and money already spent toward the end of winning rather than because of a string of independent, rational decisions.

The Dispositional Perspective

The Addictive Personality

Several theorists have noted that pathological gambling shares many features with substance use (i.e., addictive) disorders (see Chapter 4, "Categorization"). For example, both disorders often involve appetitive urges ("craving") (Castellani and Rugle 1995); the need for increased intensity of a stimulus to maintain excitement ("tolerance") (Blanco et al. 2001); and increased restlessness and irritability and decreased ability to concentrate on cessation of the activity ("withdrawal") (Wray and Dickerson 1981). Pathological gambling and substance use also frequently entail a loss of control, preoccupation with the activity, and the continued engagement in the activity despite negative consequences (Wray and Dickerson 1981). Furthermore, factors that may initially motivate individuals to either use substances or place bets include the desire to escape from an unpleasant reality or from an uncomfortable level of arousal (Wray and Dickerson 1981).

Certain personality characteristics may promote pathological gambling as well as other impulse control disorders such as substance abuse. For example, being extremely extroverted, neurotic, or impulsive increases one's risk for addictions in general (McCown and Chamberlain 2000). In one study, it was found that individuals with multiple addictions (gambling or substance use) were more impulsive than those with only one addiction (Vitaro et al. 1998).

Individuals with addictions tend to share two common features: 1) being chronically overaroused or underaroused; and 2) having experienced unfortunate experiences in childhood that led to feelings of inadequacy, rejection, or guilt (Jacobs 1986). Chronically underaroused individuals may gamble or use stimulants to reduce levels of boredom. Individuals who are chronically overaroused may cope by using depressants (e.g., alcohol). Furthermore, Martinez-Pina et al. (1991) reported that adults diagnosed with pathological gambling report frequent feelings of inferiority and rejection in childhood. Problem gamblers may have low ego strength (Livingston 1974), and playing games of skill (e.g., poker) may raise self-esteem by creating feelings of success when a person beats the odds or another player and feels admired (Lesieur 1979).

Impulsiveness

Impulsiveness can be defined as acting with little forethought, self-control, or regard for consequences. Trait impulsiveness may promote pathological gambling, and research has shown that problem gamblers score higher on measures of impulsiveness than do nongamblers, recreational gamblers, and even those addicted to alcohol or cocaine (Castellani and Rugle 1995; Steel and Blaszczynski 1998). In addition, impulsivity has been found to correlate with severity of gambling behavior among problem gamblers (Steel and Blaszczynski 1998). Among 248 male college students, those who tended to "chase" their losses were more impulsive on average than those who did not (Breen and Zuckerman 1999). Among males, impulsivity in early adolescence predicted gambling behavior several years later (Vitaro et al. 1997).

Impulsivity may lead to a loss of control when gambling. Impulsive individuals may be highly responsive to positive reinforcement but rather insensitive to punishment. Impulsive individuals may have to struggle to imagine negative outcomes (Vitaro et al. 1997). Such operant dynamics may make impulsive individuals especially vulnerable to games with rapid, intermittent payouts (e.g., slot machines). Impulsive individuals may also lack the capacity to divide attention among competing stimuli and therefore may be insensitive to internally generated cognitions focusing on restraint (McCown and Chamberlain 2000). As such, the initiation of gambling behavior may quickly lead to a loss of control. Two retrospective studies found that problem gamblers had greater attention deficits and a greater incidence of attention-deficit/hyperactivity disorder as children than did members of control groups (Carlton and Manowitz 1994; Specker et al. 1995).

Sensation Seeking

Individuals who are high in sensation seeking search for novel, exciting experiences that may entail an element of physical or social risk (Zuckerman 1979). High levels of sensation seeking have been associated with gambling (Coventry and Brown 1993) and problem gambling (Breen and Zuckerman 1999; Kuley and Jacobs 1988). Pathological gamblers score higher than social gamblers on measures of disinhibition, boredom susceptibility, and experience seeking (Dickerson et al. 1987). Individuals high in sensation seeking may seek forms of gambling that provide excitement and produce high arousal (e.g., casino gambling or illicit gambling) but may avoid other forms that do not (e.g., off-course betting) (Coventry and Brown 1993).

Extraversion

Extraverts prefer to spend time with others, especially when confronted with stress, whereas introverts prefer solitary activities (Jung 1933).

Extraverted gamblers may seek out table games, whereas introverted gamblers prefer slot machines or sports betting. Recent advancements into the biological underpinnings suggest that introversion may be a protective factor against pathological gambling, whereas extroversion may be a risk factor. For example, introverts are more aroused at baseline in limbic areas of the brain (e.g., the amygdala) and therefore are particularly sensitive to punishment (Eysenck 1983). Introverts are hypersensitive to losing money (i.e., being punished) but are hyposensitive to winning money (i.e., being rewarded) (McCown and Chamberlain 2000). Conversely, extraversion is thought to be associated with incentive (i.e., reward) sensitivity (Carver and White 1994). Furthermore, because extraverts are generally further from optimal arousal level at rest compared with introverts (Eysenck 1981), they may be more likely to seek out stimulating gambling environments to reach a comfortable level of cortical arousal. The relationship between extraversion and problem gambling, however, is complicated, with some researchers reporting a positive relationship (Bartussek et al. 1993) and others reporting no relationship (Malkin and Syme 1986).

Neuroticism

Individuals who are high in neuroticism experience negative emotions (such as feelings of nervousness, tension, or fear) more frequently than others. Measures of neuroticism may be elevated in pathological gamblers compared with nongamblers (e.g., Barnes and Parwani 1987; Roy et al. 1989), although one study failed to find elevated levels of neuroticism among young slot machine players (Carroll and Huxley 1994). No direction of causality can be inferred from these correlational studies, because theoretically both trait neuroticism and gambling behavior may promote one another. In one study prospectively examining this issue, it was found that the relationship between gambling behavior and neurotic feelings was in fact bidirectional (McCown and Chamberlain 2000). Possible reasons for a relationship between neuroticism and gambling behavior are described earlier in this chapter, in "Negative-Reinforcement Models."

Antisocial Personality Trait

Persons who are described as antisocial tend to be impulsive and high in sensation seeking, but they also disregard social convention and are apt to commit crimes. Perhaps not surprisingly, Minnesota Multiphasic Personality Inventory profiles of problem gamblers show elevation on the Psychopathic Deviant Scale (e.g., Graham and Lowenfeld 1986), which was designed to detect trait antisocial personality tendencies. The odds ratio for having antisocial personality disorder in those with gambling problems (vs. the general population) ranges from 3 (Blaszczynski and McConaghy 1994) to 6 (Cunningham-Williams et al. 1998).

The direction of effect remains unclear in the case of antisocial personality disorder. Because antisocial individuals tend to be impulsive, socially nonconforming, and risk taking, they may have an increased proclivity to gamble. Conversely, losing money through gambling may encourage antisocial acts such as writing bad checks and stealing (Blaszczynski et al. 1997). Alternatively, a third factor may promote both problems. Twin studies reveal evidence for a common genetic vulnerability for antisocial personality disorder and pathological gambling (Slutske et al. 2001).

Psychogenic Needs

Needs have been defined as internal states that are unsatisfied and therefore may guide behavior (Murray 1938). Individuals with pathological gambling may be high in the need for power (McCown and Chamberlain 2000). When gamblers were provided a moderate dose of alcohol, gambling led to fantasies about performing acts of social justice with winnings. However, when provided a high dose of alcohol, gambling led to fantasies about manifesting control over other people (McCown and Chamberlain 2000). Such fantasies may be reinforcing and may place individuals who are high in need for power at greater risk for addiction. In addition, pathological gamblers scored particularly high on the needs for achievement, exhibition, dominance, and deference (Moravec and Munley 1983).

Proclivity Toward Dissociation

Dissociation, which has been described as a trancelike state, involves the separation of normally connected mental processes. Dissociation has been seen as a possible risk factor for addictive behavior (Jacobs 1986) and may promote gambling behavior, especially among video gamblers (McCown and Chamberlain 2000). McCown and Chamberlain (2000) suggested that gamblers are relatively insensitive to disruption in gambling and that they can play for long periods of time with a reduced awareness of environmental stimuli, internal states (e.g., hunger), and time. Partners of video gamblers observed that the gamblers were more prone to dissociation while gambling than while eating or watching television.

However, other studies have produced conflicting evidence of dissociation in gamblers and may reflect the difficulty of measuring dissociation in the absence of gambling behavior, because the instruments may not account for the state-dependent characteristic of dissociation. In one study examining dissociative tendencies in various types of gamblers and in individuals with alcoholism, the researchers found that although gamblers generally were more prone toward dissociation than were individuals with alcoholism, video machine gamblers were not (Kofoed et al. 1997). However, another study showed that rates of dissociation may be no higher in subjects with pathological gambling than in healthy control subjects (Grant and Kim 2003).

Relationship of Psychological Theories to Neurobiological Systems

Operant Models

One explanation for why all individuals who gamble do not succumb to disorder-inducing intermittent reinforcement contingencies is that different win-loss patterns early in one's gambling experience may produce distinct behavioral trajectories, only some of which lead to pathological gambling. Another explanation is that individual differences in biological constraints surrounding reinforcement sensitivity might regulate response to the operant contingencies inherent in gambling. For some individuals, negative or positive reinforcement from gambling may have a more powerful influence on future gambling. Alternatively, some individuals may be more or less sensitive or responsive to the punishment associated with losses or the social opprobrium related to gambling. Searching for such individual difference-moderating variables may ultimately refine both the psychological and biological understanding of operant processes in the etiology and maintenance of pathological gambling.

Cognitive Models

The agenda of integrating cognitive theories of pathological gambling with biological processes is arguably less straightforward than in the case of operant theories because the interface between conscious thought, brain activity, and self-directed behavior is complex and incompletely understood. Does disordered thinking cause individuals to make irrational decisions and, based on these decisions, gamble pathologically? By contrast, perhaps those who are driven to gamble pathologically are prone toward confabulating ideas and views that are consistent with their behavior. Supporting the causal status of irrational thinking in promoting problem gambling are data showing that treatments aimed primarily at changing inaccurate gambling beliefs are effective in reducing pathological gambling behavior (e.g., Ladouceur et al. 1998). The apparent responsiveness of pathological gambling to cognitive interventions, however, does not unambiguously demonstrate a cognitive etiology.

A memory-based bioinformational model of pathological gambling is a particularly useful paradigm for embedding cognitive theories within generally understood biological systems. Foa and Kozak (1986) proposed a theory that fear is represented as a coherent network in memory that includes information about stimuli associated with fear, fear-based responses, and meaning (for the self) of these stimuli and responses. Basic fear-conditioning research has supported the role of memory in the acquisition and relief of fear responses and has related these processes to brain function involving protein synthesis in the lateral and basal nuclei of the amygdala (Nader et al. 2000). Similar memory structures integrated with brain systems responsible for stimuli valuation and/or appetitive behavior (as opposed to those related to fear responding) may provide a starting point in the search for a biologically grounded formulation of gambling behavior in which cognition plays a central role.

A bioinformational theory of pathological gambling provides direction for additional biopsychological research into the etiology of pathological gambling (e.g., brain systems and processes underlying activation and modification of appetitive memory structures) and provides straightforward predictions about necessary and sufficient elements of effective treatment. The latter include 1) activation of the gambling-related appetitive memory structure and 2) the incorporation of information that is incompatible with pathological elements of the memory structure. Exposure-based procedures may be the most efficient psychological approach when fear structures are involved (Foa and Kozak 1986). Although exposure-based procedures may not modify the appetitive-based structures hypothesized to drive gambling behaviors, limited data support the usefulness of exposure-based procedures in gambling (e.g., McConaghy et al. 1991). Also, based on the efficacy of cognitive therapy, education and Socratic questioning may serve to modify pathological elements of the type of memory structures proposed.

Trait or Dispositional Models

Some individuals may possess broad traits, characteristics, or response proclivities that leave them vulnerable to pathological involvement with particular classes of stimuli, including those relevant to pathological gambling. A common neurobiological process may underlie the urge to engage in a range of appetitive behaviors (Grant et al. 2002). Thus, some of the traits or dispositions purported to predispose individuals to gambling (e.g., impaired impulse control) may reflect an underlying biologically based vulnerability that includes pathological gambling. Evidence for this position includes the following: 1) neurological data implicating the ventral tegmental area/nucleus accumbens/orbital frontal cortex circuits as a potential source of an appetitive urge–based brain mechanism; 2) psychopharmacological data indicating that pathological gambling, along with a wide range of disorders related to impulse control, responds to the same medication treatments; and 3) epidemiological data demonstrating that having a pathological gambling disorder substantially increases one's risk of having a number of other impulse control disorders involving strong appetitive urges (e.g., drug and alcohol use disorders). The view that pathological gambling vulnerability is related to one or more broad psychological traits, which are themselves manifestations of a specific neurobiological status, receives substantial indirect support.

Conclusion

Psychological models provide an important perspective in understanding the etiology and maintenance of pathological gambling. We have attempted to provide an overview of the major psychological theories of pathological gambling and have argued that these models are most informative when integrated with what is known about neurobiological processes. Whether one applies a top-down or bottom-up approach, a biopsychological perspective will, we believe, provide the most useful road map for the treatment and prevention of pathological gambling.

References

Arkes HR, Ayton P: The sunk cost and Concorde effects: are humans less rational than lower animals? Psychol Bull 125:591–600, 1999

Barnes BL, Parwani S: Personality assessment of compulsive gamblers. Indian J Clin Psychol 14:98–99, 1987

Bartussek D, Diedrich O, Naumann E, et al: Introversion-extraversion and event-related potential (ERP): a test of J.A. Gray's theory. Pers Individ Dif 14:565–574, 1993

Black DW, Moyer T: Clinical features and psychiatric comorbidity of subjects with pathological gambling behavior. Psychiatr Serv 49:1434–1439, 1998

Blanco C, Moreyra P, Nunes EV, et al: Pathological gambling: addiction or compulsion? Semin Clin Neuropsychol 6:167–176, 2001

Blaszczynski A, McConaghy N: Anxiety and/or depression in the pathogenesis of addictive gambling. Int J Addict 24:337–350, 1989

Blaszczynski A, McConaghy N: Antisocial personality disorder and pathological gambling. J Gambl Stud 10:129–145, 1994

Blaszczynski A, Steel Z, McConaghy N: Impulsivity in pathological gambling: the antisocial impulsivist. Addiction 92:75–87, 1997

Breen RB, Zuckerman M: 'Chasing' in gambling behavior: personality and cognitive determinants. Pers Individ Dif 27:1097–1111, 1999

Carlton PL, Manowitz P: Factors determining the severity of pathological gambling in males. J Gambl Stud 10:147–157, 1994

Carroll D, Huxley J: Cognitive, dispositional, and psychophysiological correlates of dependent slot machine gambling in young people. J Appl Soc Sci 24:1070–1083, 1994

Carver CS, White TL: Behavioral inhibition, behavioral activation, and affective responses to impending reward and punishment: the BIS/BAS scales. J Pers Soc Psychol 67:319–333, 1994

Castellani B, Rugle L: A comparison of pathological gamblers to alcoholics and cocaine misusers on impulsivity, sensation seeking, and craving. Int J Addict 30:275–289, 1995

Cocco N, Sharpe L, Blaszczynski AP: Differences in preferred level of arousal in two sub-groups of problem gamblers: a preliminary report. J Gambl Stud 11:221–229, 1995

Coventry KR, Brown RIF: Sensation seeking, gambling and gambling addictions. Addiction 88:541–554, 1993

Coventry KR, Norman AC: Arousal, sensation seeking and frequency of gambling in off-course horse racing bettors. Br J Psychol 88:671–681, 1997

Cunningham-Williams RM, Cottler LB, Compton WM III, et al: Taking chances: problem gamblers and mental health disorders—results from the St. Louis Epidemiologic Catchment Area Study. Am J Public Health 88:1093–1096, 1998

Dickerson MG, Hinchy J, Fabre J: Chasing, arousal, and sensation seeking in off-course gamblers. Br J Addict 82:673–680, 1987

Eysenck HJ: Behavior therapy and the conditioning model of neurosis. Int J Psychol 16:343–370, 1981

Eysenck HJ: Drugs as research tools in psychology: experiments with drugs in personality research. Neuropsychobiology 10:29–43, 1983

Foa EB, Kozak MJ: Emotional processing of fear: exposure to corrective information. Psychol Bull 99:20–25, 1986

Graham JR, Lowenfeld BH: Personality dimensions of the pathological gambler. Journal of Gambling Behavior 2:58–66, 1986

Grant JE, Kim SW: Dissociative symptoms in pathological gambling. Psychopathology 36:200–203, 2003

Grant JE, Kushner MG, Kim SW: Pathological gambling and alcohol use disorder. Alcohol Res Health 26:143–150, 2002

Hayano D: Poker Faces: The Life and Work of Professional Card Players. Berkeley, CA, University of California Press, 1982

Jacobs DF: A general theory of addictions: a new theoretical model. Journal of Gambling Behavior 2:15–31, 1986

Jung C: Psychological Types. New York, Harcourt, Brace & World, 1933

Kofoed L, Morgan TJ, Buchkowski J, et al: Dissociative Experiences Scale and MMPI-2 scores in video poker gamblers, other gamblers, and alcoholic controls. J Nerv Ment Dis 185:58–60, 1997

Kuley N, Jacobs D: The relationship between dissociative-like experiences and sensation-seeking among social and problem gamblers. Journal of Gambling Behavior 4:197–207, 1988

Ladouceur R, Sylvain C, Letarte H, et al: Cognitive treatment of pathological gamblers. Behav Res Ther 36:1111–1119, 1998

Lesieur HR: The compulsive gambler's spiral of options and involvement. Psychiatry 42:79–87, 1979

Livingston J: Compulsive gamblers: a culture of losers. Psychol Today 10:51–55, 1974

Lopez Viets V, Miller W: Treatment approaches for pathological gamblers. Clin Psychol Rev 17:689–702, 1997

Malkin D, Syme G: Personality and problem gambling. Int J Addict 21:267–272, 1986

Martinez-Pina A, de Parga JLG, Vallverdu RF, et al: The Catalonia Survey: personality and intelligence structure in a sample of compulsive gamblers. J Gambl Stud 4:275–299, 1991

McCabe KA, Smith VL: A comparison of naive and sophisticated subject behavior with game theoretic predictions. Proc Natl Acad Sci USA 97:3777–3781, 2000

McConaghy N: Behavior completion mechanisms rather than primary drives maintain behavioral patterns. Act Nerv Super (Praha) 22:138–151, 1980

McConaghy N, Blaszczynski A, Frankova A: Comparison of imaginal desensitisation with other behavioural treatments of pathological gambling: a two- to nine-year follow-up. Br J Psychiatry 159:390–393, 1991

McCown WG, Chamberlain LL: Best Possible Odds: Contemporary Treatment Strategies for Gambling Disorders. New York, Wiley, 2000

Moravec JD, Munley PH: Psychological test findings on pathological gamblers. Int J Addict 18:1003–1009, 1983

Murray H: Explorations in Personality. New York, Oxford University Press, 1938

Nader K, Schafe GE, Le Doux JE: Fear memories require protein synthesis in the amygdala for reconsolidation after retrieval. Nature 406:722–726, 2000

Ocean G, Smith GJ: Social reward, conflict, and commitment: a theoretical model of gambling behavior. J Gambl Stud 9:321–329, 1993

Rogers P: The cognitive psychology of lottery gambling: a theoretical review. J Gambl Stud 14:111–134, 1998

Roy A, Custer R, Lorenz V, et al: Personality factors and pathological gambling. Acta Psychiatr Scand 80:37–39, 1989

Sharpe L: A reformulated cognitive-behavioral model of problem gambling. A biopsychosocial perspective. Clin Psychol Rev 22:1–25, 2002

Slutske WS, Eisen S, Xian H, et al: A twin study of the association between pathological gambling and antisocial personality disorder. J Abnorm Psychol 110:297–308, 2001

Snyder W: Decision-making with risk and uncertainty: the case of horse racing. Am J Psychol 91:201–209, 1978

Specker SM, Carlson GA, Christenson GA, et al: Impulse control disorders and attention deficit disorder in pathological gamblers. Ann Clin Psychiatry 7:175–179, 1995

Steel Z, Blaszczynski A: Impulsivity, personality disorders and pathological gambling severity. Addiction 93:895–905, 1998

Toneatto T: Cognitive psychopathology of problem gambling. Subst Use Misuse 34:1593–1604, 1999

Tversky A, Kahneman D: The framing of decisions and the psychology of choice. Science 211:453–458, 1981

Vitaro F, Arsenault L, Tremblay RE: Dispositional predictors of problem gambling in male adolescents. Am J Psychiatry 154:1769–1770, 1997

Vitaro F, Ferland F, Jacques C, et al: Gambling, substance use, and impulsivity during adolescence. Psychol Addict Behav 12:185–194, 1998

Walker MB: Irrational thinking among slot machine players. J Gambl Stud 8:245–261, 1992

Wray I, Dickerson MG: Cessation of high frequency gambling and "withdrawal" symptoms. Br J Addict 76:401–405, 1981

Zuckerman M: Sensation Seeking: Beyond the Optimal Level of Arousal. Hillsdale, NJ, Erlbaum, 1979

Biological Basis for Pathological Gambling

Kamini R. Shah, M.H.S.
Marc N. Potenza, M.D., Ph.D.
Seth A. Eisen, M.D.

Research into the biology of pathological gambling is in an early stage (Eber and Shaffer 2000). Mounting data suggest that multiple neurotransmitter systems are involved in the pathophysiology of pathological gambling (Potenza 2001). In this chapter we review evidence that supports the involvement of the noradrenergic, serotonergic, dopaminergic, and opioidergic systems, and familial and inherited factors in pathological gambling.

Neurobiology

Serotonergic Mechanisms

The most fully documented neurobiological findings regarding impulse control disorders involve serotonin (5-hydroxyindole or 5-hydroxytryptamine [5-HT]) (Potenza 2001). Evidence for involvement of 5-HT in pathological gambling (Table 9–1) comes from studies of platelet activity of monoamine oxidase B (MAO B), a peripheral marker of 5-HT function (Ibáñez et al. 2002). Low cerebrospinal fluid (CSF) levels of the

5-HT metabolite 5-hydroxyindoleacetic acid—correlating with high levels of impulsivity (Oreland et al. 1998) and sensation seeking (Ward et al. 1987)—or low MAO B platelet activity, or both, have been found in three studies of pathological gamblers (Blanco et al. 1996; Carrasco et al. 1994; Nordin and Eklundh 1999), but not in two others (Bergh et al. 1997; Roy et al. 1988). In two studies in which lower platelet MAO activity was found in pathological gamblers (Blanco et al. 1996), the previously reported association between low platelet MAO activity and sensation seeking was not present among the pathological gamblers. Therefore, the relationship between 5-HT function and impulsiveness and sensation seeking in pathological gambling requires further study.

Pharmacological challenge studies also provide evidence for serotonergic dysfunction in pathological gambling. Blunted prolactin release was observed in pathological gamblers compared with control subjects in response to a single intravenous dose (12.5 mg) of clomipramine, a serotonin reuptake inhibitor (DeCaria et al. 1998). Another study demonstrated increased prolactin response to a single oral dose (0.5 mg/kg) of *m*-chlorophenylpiperazine (a partial 5-HT_1 and 5-HT_2 agonist) in male pathological gamblers compared with healthy volunteers, a finding consistent with 5-HT postsynaptic receptor hypersensitivity and decreased 5-HT availability (DeCaria et al. 1998). Additional support for serotonergic involvement in pathological gambling comes from double-blind, placebo-controlled treatment trials of clomipramine, fluvoxamine, and paroxetine, although not all studies have demonstrated positive results (see Chapter 13, "Pharmacological Treatments"). Together, these studies implicate the 5-HT system in pathological gambling, indicate a complex relationship between 5-HT and pathological gambling, and suggest that further research is needed to understand the specific mechanisms involved.

Dopaminergic Mechanisms

The dopaminergic mesocortical limbic system, believed to underlie reward and reinforcement in healthy and disordered states, has been implicated in pathological gambling (Table 9–1) (Potenza et al. 2001). Multiple lines of evidence suggest that rewarding and reinforcing behaviors result in dopamine release from dopaminergic cells in the ventral tegmental area into the nucleus accumbens (Comings and Blum 2000).

Age-related changes in dopaminergic system function have been implicated in gambling and pathological gambling. One model proposes that changes in dopaminergic and 5-HT function during adolescence may underlie adolescent vulnerability to gambling problems (Chambers and Potenza 2003). Older adults, a group with diminished dopaminergic

Table 9–1. Neurotransmitter systems implicated in the pathophysiology of pathological gambling

Neurotransmitter	Proposed role	Supporting data
Norepinephrine (NE)	Arousal, excitement	Elevated urinary levels of NE and cerebrospinal fluid (CSF) levels of the NE metabolite 3-methoxy-4-hydroxyphenylglycol (MHPG) in men with pathological gambling (Roy et al. 1988, 1989b); elevated CSF levels of NE and MHPG in men with pathological gambling (Bergh et al. 1997), but not after correcting for CSF flow rates (Nordin and Eklundh 1999)
Serotonin (5-HT)	Impulse control	Abnormal biochemical and behavioral responses to serotonergic drugs clomipramine and *m*-chlorophenylpiperazine (DeCaria et al. 1998); decreased CSF levels of 5-HT metabolite 5-hydroxyindoleacetic acid (Nordin and Eklundh 1999); decreased platelet monoamine oxidase (MAO) activity in men with pathological gambling (Blanco et al. 1996; Carrasco et al. 1994); efficacy of selective serotonin reuptake inhibitors in the treatment of pathological gambling (see Chapter 12, "Cognitive and Behavioral Treatments"); short allele of 5-HT transporter gene found more frequently in men with pathological gambling (reviewed in Ibáñez et al. 2003); 3-repeat allele of MAO A promoter allele found more frequently in men with pathological gambling (reviewed in Ibáñez et al. 2003)
Dopamine	Reward, reinforcement	Decreased CSF levels of dopamine and increased levels of dopamine metabolites in men with pathological gambling (Bergh et al. 1997), not seen when correcting for CSF flow rates (Nordin and Eklundh 1999); 7-repeat allele of dopamine D_4 receptor gene (*DRD4*) found more frequently in women with pathological gambling (reviewed in Ibáñez et al. 2003)
Opioids	Pleasure, urges	Efficacy of μ opioid receptor antagonist naltrexone in the treatment of pathological gambling (see Chapter 12, "Cognitive and Behavioral Treatments")

function, demonstrate lower rates of gambling and pathological gambling (see Chapter 6, "Older Adults"). However, the observation of onset or worsening of pathological gambling in older individuals with Parkinson's disease after the initial administration of pro-dopaminergic drugs suggests that increased dopaminergic function in part leads to pathological gambling (Gschwandtner et al. 2001; Molina et al. 2000; Seedat et al. 2000).

Other investigations of dopaminergic system dysregulation in pathological gambling provide mixed results. Comparisons of the CSF of male pathological gamblers and control subjects have found decreased dopamine levels and increased dopamine metabolites in the pathological gambling group, a finding suggestive of increased dopamine turnover (Bergh et al. 1997). However, this difference was not observed when correcting for CSF flow rates (Nordin and Eklundh 1999). Another study found no differences in plasma, urinary, or CSF dopamine levels between subjects with pathological gambling and unaffected subjects (Roy et al. 1988). More positive findings suggestive of dopaminergic involvement in gambling behaviors come from studies of healthy subjects during gambling-like behaviors. Koepp and colleagues (1998) reported increased striatal dopamine release in males playing a tank video game for money. Healthy subjects displayed increased activity in the ventral tegmental area and its projection sites during viewing of a spinner that could land on regions of a circle corresponding to good, bad, or intermediate monetary values (Breiter et al. 2001). The extent of the differences between subjects with pathological gambling and control subjects that occur during performance of these tasks requires further investigation.

Noradrenergic Mechanisms

Noradrenergic systems—believed to underlie arousal, excitement, and sensation seeking—have been implicated in pathological gambling (Table 9–1). Gambling produces increased autonomic activation in pathological gambling (Leary and Dickerson 1985). Urinary noradrenergic output and CSF concentrations of noradrenaline and 3-methoxy-4-hydroxyphenylglycol (a noradrenergic metabolite) were found to be higher in pathological gambling subjects than in control subjects (Bergh et al. 1997; Roy et al. 1988). Extraversion correlated with markers of noradrenergic function, which suggested that central noradrenergic functioning in pathological gambling influences personality (Roy et al. 1989b). A challenge study found enhanced growth hormone response to clonidine (0.15 mg), an α_2-adrenergic agonist, in pathological gambling, and a dose-response relationship existed between the growth hormone response and severity of illness (DeCaria et al. 1998).

Opioidergic Mechanisms

The μ opioid system is believed to underlie urge regulation through the processing of reward, pleasure, and pain—at least in part via modulation of dopamine neurons in the mesolimbic pathway through γ-aminobutyric acid (GABA) interneurons (Broekkamp and Phillips 1979)—and has been hypothesized as mediating aspects of pathological gambling (Table 9–1). The μ opioid receptor is the site at which β-endorphins, morphine, and heroin act as agonists. The μ opioid system has been linked to physiological responses during the gambling-like activity pachinko (Shinohara et al. 1999). Although a separate study found similar CSF levels of β-endorphin in subjects with pathological gambling and control subjects, lower levels were observed in pathological gamblers who bet on horse races compared with those who bet by using slot machines, suggesting the existence of biologically relevant differences based on types of gambling (Blaszczynski et al. 1986).

Additional support for opioidergic involvement in pathological gambling comes from studies of naltrexone, a drug that is effective in the treatment of alcohol dependence (O'Malley et al. 1992; Volpicelli et al. 1992) and opioid dependence (Hollister et al. 1977). Naltrexone, a μ opioid receptor antagonist, was found to be superior to placebo in the short-term treatment of pathological gambling, particularly in those who experience strong urges to gamble (see Chapter 13, "Pharmacological Treatments").

Brain Imaging Studies

Few brain imaging studies in pathological gambling have been performed. A functional magnetic resonance imaging (fMRI) study of gambling urges in male pathological gamblers suggests that pathological gambling has neural features similar to those of other impulse control disorders and distinct from those of obsessive-compulsive disorder (Potenza et al. 2003b). During the initial presentation of gambling cues, pathological gamblers displayed relative decreases in activity within cortical, basal ganglionic, and thalamic brain regions compared with control subjects. In contrast, increased cortico-basal-ganglionic-thalamic activity has been observed in obsessive-compulsive disorder (Saxena and Rauch 2000). During the most provocative gambling stimuli, pathological gamblers showed relatively decreased activity in the ventromedial prefrontal cortex, a brain region implicated in decision making and impulse control (Bechara 2003; Best et al. 2002; New et al. 2002). An independent fMRI Stroop Test (color-word interference task) investigation of males with pathological gambling also found relatively decreased ventromedial prefrontal cortical activity in pathological gambling (Potenza et al. 2003a). Taken together, these data suggest that pathological gambling shares similar neural features with other disorders or conditions characterized by impaired impulse control.

Neurocognitive Studies

A comparison of non-substance-abusing gamblers with nonaddicted control subjects showed that problem gamblers had more childhood behaviors consistent with attention deficits and demonstrated poorer performance on higher-order attention measures (Rugle and Melamed 1993). Male and female pathological gamblers had slower reactions than occasional gamblers to irrelevant external light stimuli when gambling at a video lottery terminal machine, suggesting that pathological gamblers experience a greater narrowing of attention than do occasional gamblers during video lottery terminal gambling (Diskin and Hodgins 1999). Poker machine gamblers who experienced difficulty controlling their gambling behavior took significantly longer than gamblers with good control to name the colors of the words relating to poker machine gambling (but not those of neutral or drug-related words) in a gambling-specific Stroop interference task (Boyer and Dickerson 2003).

Compared with healthy control subjects, pathological gamblers tend to place a greater salience on immediate rewards as assessed by measures of temporal discounting or a gambling task (Cavedini et al. 2002a; Petry 2001a, 2001b; Petry and Casarella 1999). The gambling task simulates real-life decision making and tests the ability to make advantageous decisions by balancing immediate and delayed rewards and punishments (Bechara 2003). The disadvantageous decision making, thought to involve ventromedial prefrontal cortical function, was similar to that of individuals with drug addiction (Bechara 2003) or obsessive-compulsive disorder (Cavedini et al. 2002b).

Other Biological Associations

Arousal and Stress

Multiple studies have found increased heart rate, blood pressure, and cortisol release during gambling. Gamblers demonstrated elevated heart rates while gambling at casinos, off-track betting locations, and video terminals (Anderson and Brown 1984; Coventry and Norman 1997; Leary and Dickerson 1985). Habitual male gamblers demonstrated increased salivary cortisol levels and heart rates during casino blackjack gambling (Meyer et al. 2000). Another investigation found autonomic arousal to be differentially elevated based on biological indicators (skin conductance level, heart rate, frontalis electromyography), the type of gambler (problem, low frequency, and high frequency), and experimental condition (Sharpe et al. 1995). Autonomic arousal (norepinephrine levels, heart rate) and immune system changes have been documented in habitual male pachinko players (Shinohara et al. 1999), and higher epinephrine and cortisol levels were found in an Aboriginal group on days in which gambling was concentrated (Schmitt et al. 1998). Gambling-related stimuli were associated with increases in arousal that were greatest for problem gamblers, even in the absence of apparent differences in behavior (Sharpe et al. 1995). Together, these findings suggest that gambling across nonproblematic and pathological gambling groups represents a mildly stressful experience involving alterations in stress hormones, adrenergic function, and physiological measures.

Electroencephalographic Studies

Men with a history of pathological gambling and matched nongambler control subjects underwent electroencephalographic recordings of brain activity during tasks designed to differentially and successively activate the left (verbal) and right (visual) cerebral hemispheres. These recordings indicated that shifts in laterality were minimal for gamblers and took longer to become established when they did occur (Goldstein and Carlton 1988). The decreased shifts in laterality may reflect a compulsive feature of pathological gambling.

Cerebrospinal Fluid Studies

Nordin and Eklundh (1996) hypothesized that subjects with pathological gambling and control subjects would differ in inhibitory neurotransmitter function as reflected in CSF levels. Low levels of the inhibitory amino acid taurine were found in male pathological gamblers compared with control subjects (Nordin and Eklundh 1996). Differences in CSF levels of GABA, another inhibitory neurotransmitter, were not observed (Roy et al. 1989a).

Genetic Studies

Family Studies

Approximately 20% of pathological gamblers have first-degree relatives who also have pathological gambling (Ibáñez et al. 2002). In a study of predominantly white male Veterans Administration hospital patients, problem gamblers were 3–8 times more likely than gamblers without problems to report having at least one parent with a history of problem gambling (Gambino et al. 1993). Pathological gambling was 3 times more likely to occur among patients who perceived that their parents had gambling problems and was 12 times more likely if the patients also perceived that their grandparents had gambling problems. Among a random sample of adolescents, those who reported that their parents were pathological gamblers were more likely to be moderate to heavy gamblers and to experience negative consequences related to their gambling (Jacobs et al. 1989).

A meta-analysis of 17 family studies revealed stronger familial effects for the sons of men with problem gambling than among the daughters of women with problem gambling, and for more severe forms of problem gambling compared with less severe forms of problem wagering (Walters 2001). The strongest familial influence was found for high-severity problem gambling in males. Familial patterns have also been reported among college students who were problem gamblers (Winters et al. 1998).

Twin Studies

Twin studies permit the risk for pathological gambling to be separated into genetic, shared environmental, and nonshared environmental components (Shah et al., in press). In a study of 3,359 male-male twin pairs of the Vietnam Era Twin Registry (Henderson et al. 1990), Eisen et al. (1998) found that genes explained 35%, 48%, and 54% of the variance in the number of pathological gambling symptoms reported for no, one or more, or two or more symptoms, respectively. Familial factors explained 56% of the variance in the reporting of three or more symptoms (i.e., DSM-III-R [American Psychiatric Association 1987] pathological gambling symptoms) and 62% of the variance in the reporting of four or more symptoms. Because of small sample size, the genetic contribution to pathological gambling could not be adequately determined.

Additional analyses revealed a common genetic vulnerability between lifetime pathological gambling and two other psychiatric disorders: antisocial personality disorder (ASPD) (Slutske et al. 2001) and alcohol dependence (Slutske et al. 2000). These studies showed that 16% of the genetic and 9% of the nonshared environmental risk for pathological gambling overlapped with ASPD. Twelve percent of the genetic and 8% of the nonshared environmental risk for pathological gambling overlapped with alcohol dependence. Importantly, studies of this cohort suggest that differing severities of gambling problems fall along a continuum rather than forming distinct entities and that they share many, if not all, of the same risk factors (Shah 2002; Slutske et al. 2000).

These findings indicate that familial factors explain a substantial portion of the risk for pathological gambling and that a small but significant portion of risk for pathological gambling is accounted for by shared genetic vulnerability with alcohol dependence and ASPD. Antisocial behavior observed in persons with pathological gambling is thus not simply a consequence of their gambling. Although alcohol dependence and ASPD are both related to impulsivity and both share genetic risk factors with pathological gambling, most of the risk for pathological gambling is not explained by shared vulnerability with alcohol dependence or ASPD. These results are consistent with 1) those of a smaller study of male twins that found a significant and moderate heritability effect for high-action gambling (i.e., gambling in casinos) (Winters and Rich 1998); 2) those of a study of identical twins reared apart that provided evidence for the heritability of impulsiveness (Tellegen et al. 1988); and 3) increasing evidence that addictions have common as well as distinct neurobiological pathways (Enoch and Goldman 1999).

Molecular Genetics

Although twin studies provide estimates of the overall genetic risk for pathological gambling, they do not identify specific genes. The association of impulsive, compulsive, and addictive disorders with pathological gambling, combined with growing evidence about the role of serotonergic and dopaminergic systems in pathological gambling and the influence of genetic factors in chemical addictions (Blum et al. 1995; Tsuang et al. 1996), has focused the search for candidate genes for pathological gambling on genes that have known associations with impulsive and addictive disorders. As such, association studies in pathological gambling have focused predominantly on genes related to 5-HT and dopaminergic function.

The gene encoding MAO A, an enzyme expressed in the brain mainly in dopamine neurons, has been implicated in pathological gambling (Ibáñez et al. 2003). Specifically, an allele of the MAO A promoter associated with lower transcriptional and enzymatic activity has been found to be differentially associated with severe pathological gambling in males (Ibáñez et al. 2003). Although low levels of MAO B activity have been associated with pathological gambling (Carrasco et al. 1994), no association between an MAO B polymorphic marker and pathological gambling was found (Ibáñez et al. 2003). The less functional (short) variant of a polymorphism of the 5-HT transporter gene *(SLC6A4)*, associated with decreased promoter activity, is found more frequently in male pathological gamblers compared with control subjects (Ibáñez et al. 2003).

The Taq-A1 allele *(D2A1)* of the dopamine D_2 receptor gene *(DRD2)*—a variant associated with a variety of addictive, compulsive, and impulsive behaviors (Noble 2000)—was present in more than 50% of white pathological gamblers versus 26% of nonaddicted control subjects (Comings et al. 1996). The presence of the *D2A1* allele was related to severity of pathological gambling and was found more frequently in pathological gamblers who also met criteria for a substance use disorder (61%) than in those who did not (44%) (Comings et al. 1996). Carriers of the *DRD2* receptor A1 allele have demonstrated altered dopaminergic system function and are thought to be at risk for multiple addictive, impulsive, and compulsive disorders (Noble 2000).

The dopamine D_4 receptor gene *(DRD4)*, one inconsistently associated with novelty seeking (Benjamin et al. 1995; Malhotra et al. 1996), has been implicated in pathological gambling through a less efficient variant of a functional polymorphism (Ibáñez et al. 2003) and with heterozygosity versus homozygosity for alleles involving repeats of a 48–base pair sequence (Comings et al. 1999). Variants in the dopamine D_1 receptor gene *(DRD1)* have been reported in association with substance abuse and addictive behaviors, with one study finding an association between increased homozygosity for the *DRD1* Dde I 1 or 2 alleles and compulsive or addictive behaviors, including pathological gambling (Comings et al. 1997).

A study of 139 pathological gamblers and 139 age-, race-, and sex-matched control subjects found that polymorphisms at 15 of 31 candidate genes affected the risk for pathological gambling (Comings et al. 2001). Based on multivariate regression analysis, the genes contributing most significantly were *DRD2*, *DRD4*, dopamine transporter gene *(DAT1)*, tryptophan hydroxylase gene *(TPH)*, α_2C-adrenergic receptor gene *(ADRA2C)*, N-methyl-D-aspartate receptor gene *(NMDA1)*, and PS-1 gene *(PS1)*. Each gene accounted for only a small portion of the variation in risk for pathological gambling (i.e., less than 2% for most genes), with dopamine, 5-HT, and norepinephrine genes contributing approximately equally to the risk for pathological gambling.

Gender Differences

Most research has involved solely or predominantly males, and studies that include women have raised the possibility that important gender differences exist (Potenza et al. 2001). Preliminary findings, some of which are based on small samples, include differences in the distribution of allelic variants in the dopamine D_4 receptor and 5-HT transporter gene regions among male and female pathological gamblers (Ibáñez et al. 2003), increased frequency of the *SLC6A4* gene allele in male but not female pathological gamblers (Ibáñez et al. 2003), the association of the *DRD4–7* repeat allele with pathological gambling in women but not men (Ibáñez et al. 2003), the association for males but not females between pathological gambling and the overall allele distribution for an *MAOA* gene polymorphism (Ibáñez et al. 2003), the association of zygosity and types of gambling among men but not among women (Winters and Rich 1998), and the suggestion that fluvoxamine is superior to placebo in the treatment of male but not female pathological gamblers (Blanco et al. 2002). It has been proposed that serotonergic dysfunction might be more important in the pathophysiology of pathological gambling in men and dopaminergic dysregulation might play a larger role in women (Ibáñez et al. 2002), and that the differences in genetic influences might be related to clinical manifestations of gender differences (e.g., types and progression of gambling problems [Potenza et al. 2001; Tavares et al. 2001]).

Conclusion

Existing evidence from neurobiological, pharmacological, neuroimaging, neuropsychological, and genetic studies suggests that pathological gambling shares characteristics with substance use and impulse control disorders (Chambers and Potenza 2003; Potenza 2001). This growing body of evidence supports the role of multiple neurotransmitter systems (i.e., serotonergic, dopaminergic, noradrenergic, opioidergic) in pathological gambling. These data allow for the generation of models that can be used as the foundation for future investigations into the neurobiology of pathological gambling. For example, a model incorporating impaired frontal cortical inhibitory mechanisms, largely serotonergic in nature, and increased promotivational drive, largely dopaminergic in nature, has been proposed as underlying increased vulnerability to addictive processes (Chambers et al. 2003). More research is needed to examine the extent to which this model holds true for specific disorders at different neurodevelopmental stages and to identify and better characterize the underlying molecular, cellular, and neural processes. For example, although twin studies provide strong evidence for genetic and environmental contributions to pathological gambling, many specific aspects of the etiology of pathological gambling, including the precise role of individual genes, remain largely unknown.

References

American Psychiatric Association: Diagnostic and Statistical Manual of Mental Disorders, 3rd Edition, Revised. Washington, DC, American Psychiatric Association, 1987

Anderson G, Brown R: Real and laboratory gambling, sensation-seeking and arousal. Br J Psychol 75:401–410, 1984

Bechara A: Risky business: emotion, decision-making and addiction. J Gambl Stud 19:23–51, 2003

Benjamin J, Paterson C, Greenberg B, et al: Dopamine D4 receptor gene association with normal personality traits (letter). Psychiatr Genet 5 (suppl):S36, 1995

Bergh C, Eklund T, Sodersten P, et al: Altered dopamine function in pathological gambling. Psychol Med 27:473–475, 1997

Best M, Williams JM, Coccaro EF: Evidence for a dysfunctional prefrontal circuit in patients with an impulsive aggressive disorder. Proc Natl Acad Sci U S A 99:8448–8453, 2002

Blanco C, Orensanz-Munoz L, Blanco-Jerez C, et al: Pathological gambling and platelet MAO activity: a psychobiological study. Am J Psychiatry 153:119–121, 1996

Blanco C, Petkova E, Ibáñez A, et al: A pilot placebo-controlled study of fluvoxamine for pathological gambling. Ann Clin Psychiatry 14:9–15, 2002

Blaszczynski AP, Winter SW, McConaghy N: Plasma endorphin levels in pathological gamblers. Journal of Gambling Behavior 2:3–14, 1986

Blum K, Sheridan PJ, Wood RC, et al: Dopamine D2 receptor gene variants: association and linkage studies in impulsive-addictive-compulsive behavior. Pharmacogenetics 5:121–141, 1995

Boyer M, Dickerson M: Attentional bias and addictive behaviour: automaticity in a gambling-specific modified Stroop task. Addiction 98:61–70, 2003

Breiter HC, Aharon I, Kahneman D, et al: Functional imaging of neural responses to expectancy and experience of monetary gains and losses. Neuron 30:619–639, 2001

Broekkamp CL, Phillips AG: Facilitation of self-stimulation behavior following intracerebral microinjections of opioids into the ventral tegmental area. Pharmacol Biochem Behav 11:289–295, 1979

Carrasco JL, Saiz-Ruiz J, Hollander E, et al: Low platelet monoamine oxidase activity in pathological gambling. Acta Psychiatr Scand 90:427–431, 1994

Cavedini P, Riboldi G, D'Annucci A, et al: Decision-making heterogeneity in obsessive-compulsive disorder: ventromedial prefrontal cortex function predicts different treatment outcomes. Neuropsychologia 40:205–211, 2002a

Cavedini P, Riboldi G, Keller R, et al: Frontal lobe dysfunction in pathological gambling patients. Biol Psychiatry 51:334–341, 2002b

Chambers RA, Potenza MN: Neurodevelopment, impulsivity and adolescent gambling. J Gambl Stud 19:53–84, 2003

Chambers RA, Taylor JR, Potenza MN: Developmental neurocircuitry of motivation in adolescence: a critical period of addiction vulnerability. Am J Psychiatry 160:1041–1052, 2003

Comings DE, Blum K: Reward deficiency syndrome: genetic aspects of behavioral disorders. Prog Brain Res 126:325–341, 2000

Comings DE, Rosenthal RJ, Lesieur HR, et al: A study of the dopamine D2 receptor gene in pathological gambling. Pharmacogenetics 6:223–234, 1996

Comings DE, Gade R, Wu S, et al: Studies of the potential role of the dopamine D1 receptor gene in addictive behaviors. Mol Psychiatry 2:44–56, 1997

Comings DE, Gonzalez N, Wu S, et al: Studies of the 48 bp repeat polymorphism of the DRD4 gene in impulsive, compulsive, addictive behaviors: Tourette syndrome, ADHD, pathological gambling, and substance abuse. Am J Med Genet 88:358–368, 1999

Comings DE, Gade-Andavolu R, Gonzalez N, et al: The additive effect of neurotransmitter genes in pathological gambling. Clin Genet 60:107–116, 2001

Coventry KR, Norman AC: Arousal, sensation seeking and frequency of gambling in off-course horse racing bettors. Br J Psychol 88:671–681, 1997

DeCaria CM, Begaz T, Hollander E: Serotonergic and noradrenergic function in pathological gambling. CNS Spectr 3:38–47, 1998

Diskin KM, Hodgins DC: Narrowing of attention and dissociation in pathological video lottery gamblers. J Gambl Stud 15:17–28, 1999

Eber GB, Shaffer HJ: Trends in bio-behavioral gambling studies research: quantifying citations. J Gambl Stud 16:461–467, 2000

Eisen SA, Lin N, Lyons MJ, et al: Familial influences on gambling behavior: an analysis of 3359 twin pairs. Addiction 93:1375–1384, 1998

Enoch MA, Goldman D: Genetics of alcoholism and substance abuse. Psychiatr Clin North Am 22:289–299, 1999

Gambino B, Fitzgerald R, Shaffer HJ, et al: Perceived family history of problem gambling and scores on the SOGS. J Gambl Stud 9:169–184, 1993

Goldstein L, Carlton PL: Hemispheric EEG correlates of compulsive behavior: the case of pathological gamblers. Res Commun Psychol Psychiatr Behav 13:103–111, 1988

Gschwandtner U, Aston J, Renaud S, et al: Pathologic gambling in patients with Parkinson's disease. Clin Neuropharmacol 24:170–172, 2001

Henderson WG, Eisen S, Goldberg J, et al: The Vietnam Era Twin Registry: a resource for medical research. Public Health Rep 105:368–373, 1990

Hollister E, Schwin RL, Kasper P: Naltrexone treatment of opiate-dependent persons. Drug Alcohol Depend 2:203–209, 1977

Ibáñez A, Blanco C, Saiz-Ruiz J: Neurobiology and genetics of pathological gambling. Psychiatr Ann 32:181–185, 2002

Ibáñez A, Blanco C, de Castro IP, et al: Genetics of pathological gambling. J Gambl Stud 19:11–22, 2003

Jacobs DF, Marston AR, Singer RD, et al: Children of problem gamblers. Journal of Gambling Behavior 5:261–268, 1989

Koepp MJ, Gunn RN, Lawrence AD, et al: Evidence for striatal dopamine release during a video game. Nature 393:266–268, 1998

Leary K, Dickerson M: Levels of arousal in high- and low-frequency gamblers. Behav Res Ther 23:635–640, 1985

Malhotra AK, Virkkunen M, Rooney W, et al: The association between the dopamine D4 receptor (DRD4) 16 amino acid repeat polymorphisms and novelty seeking. Mol Psychiatry 1:388–391, 1996

Meyer G, Hauffa BP, Schedlowski M, et al: Casino gambling increases heart rate and salivary cortisol in regular gamblers. Biol Psychiatry 48:948–953, 2000

Molina JA, Sainz-Artiga MJ, Fraile A, et al: Pathologic gambling in Parkinson's disease: a behavioral manifestation of pharmacologic treatment? Mov Disord 15:869–872, 2000

New AS, Hazlett EA, Buchsbaum MS, et al: Blunted prefrontal cortical 18-fluorodeoxyglucose positron emission tomography response to meta-chlorophenylpiperazine in impulsive aggression. Arch Gen Psychiatry 59:621–629, 2002

Noble EP: Addiction and its reward process through polymorphisms of the D2 dopamine receptor gene: a review. Eur Psychiatry 15:79–89, 2000

Nordin C, Eklundh T: Lower CSF taurine levels in male pathological gamblers than in healthy controls. Hum Psychopharmacol 11:401–403, 1996

Nordin C, Eklundh T: Altered CSF 5-HIAA disposition in pathological male gamblers. CNS Spectr 4:25–33, 1999

O'Malley SS, Jaffe AJ, Chang G, et al: Naltrexone and coping skills therapy for alcohol dependence: a controlled study. Arch Gen Psychiatry 49:881–887, 1992

Oreland L, Ekblom J, Garpenstrand H, et al: Biological markers, with special regard to platelet monoamine oxidase (trbc-MAO), for personality and personality disorders. Adv Pharmacol 42:301–304, 1998

Petry NM: Pathological gamblers, with and without substance use disorders, discount delayed rewards at high rates. J Abnorm Psychol 110:482–487, 2001a

Petry NM: Substance abuse, pathological gambling, and impulsiveness. Drug Alcohol Depend 63:29–38, 2001b

Petry NM, Casarella T: Excessive discounting of delayed rewards in substance abusers with gambling problems. Drug Alcohol Depend 56:25–32, 1999

Potenza MN: The neurobiology of pathological gambling. Semin Clin Neuropsychiatry 6:217–226, 2001

Potenza MN, Steinberg MA, McLaughlin SD, et al: Gender-related differences in the characteristics of problem gamblers using a gambling helpline. Am J Psychiatry 158:1500–1505, 2001

Potenza MN, Leung H-C, Blumberg HP, et al: An event-related fMRI Stroop study of pathological gamblers. Biol Psychiatry 53:54S, 2003a

Potenza MN, Steinberg MA, Skudlarski P, et al: An fMRI study of gambling urges in pathological gamblers. Arch Gen Psychiatry 60:828–836, 2003b

Roy A, Adinoff B, Roehrich L, et al: Pathological gambling: a psychobiological study. Arch Gen Psychiatry 45:369–373, 1988

Roy A, DeJong J, Ferraro T, et al: CSF GABA and neuropeptides in pathological gamblers and normal controls. Psychiatr Res 30:137–144, 1989a

Roy A, De Jong J, Linnoila M: Extraversion in pathological gamblers: correlates with indexes of noradrenergic function. Arch Gen Psychiatry 46:679–681, 1989b

Rugle L, Melamed L: Neuropsychological assessment of attention problems in pathological gamblers. J Nerv Ment Dis 181:107–112, 1993

Saxena S, Rauch SL: Functional neuroimaging and the neuroanatomy of obsessive-compulsive disorder. Psychiatr Clin North Am 23:1–19, 2000

Schmitt LH, Harrison GA, Spargo RM: Variation in epinephrine and cortisol excretion rates associated with behavior in an Australian Aboriginal community. Am J Phys Anthropol 106:249–253, 1998

Seedat S, Kesler S, Niehaus DJH, et al: Pathological gambling behaviour: emergence secondary to treatment of Parkinson's disease with dopaminergic agents. Depress Anxiety 11:185–186, 2000

Shah KR: A latent class typology of gambling behaviors in a population-based sample. Paper presented at the 16th National Conference on Problem Gambling, National Council on Problem Gambling, Dallas, TX. June 14, 2002

Shah KR, Eisen SE, Xian H, et al: Genetic studies of pathological gambling: a review of methodology and analyses of data from the Vietnam Era Twin (VET) Registry. J Gambl Stud (in press)

Sharpe L, Tarrier N, Schotte D, et al: The role of autonomic gambling arousal in problem gambling. Addiction 90:1529–1540, 1995

Shinohara K, Yanagisawa A, Kagota Y, et al: Physiological changes in Pachinko players; beta-endorphin, catecholamines, immune system substances and heart rate. Appl Human Sci 18:37–42, 1999

Slutske WS, Eisen S, True WR, et al: Common genetic vulnerability for pathological gambling and alcohol dependence in men. Arch Gen Psychiatry 57:666–673, 2000

Slutske WS, Eisen S, Xian H, et al: A twin study of the association between pathological gambling and antisocial personality disorder. J Abnorm Psychol 110:297–308, 2001

Tavares H, Zilberman ML, Beites FJ, et al: Gender differences in gambling progression. J Gambl Stud 17:151–159, 2001

Tellegen A, Lykken DT, Bouchard TJ, et al: Personality similarity in twins reared apart and together. J Pers Soc Psychol 54:1031–1039, 1988

Tsuang MT, Lyons MJ, Eisen SA, et al: Genetic influences on DSM-III-R drug abuse and dependence: a study of 3,372 twin pairs. Am J Med Genet 67:473–477, 1996

Volpicelli JR, Alterman AI, Hayashida M, et al: Naltrexone in the treatment of alcohol dependence. Arch Gen Psychiatry 49:876–880, 1992

Walters GD: Behavior genetic research on gambling and problem gambling: a preliminary meta-analysis of available data. J Gambl Stud 17:255–271, 2001

Ward PB, Catts SV, Norman TR, et al: Low platelet monoamine oxidase and sensation seeking in males: an established relationship? Acta Psychiatr Scand 75:86–90, 1987

Winters KC, Rich T: A twin study of adult gambling behavior. J Gambl Stud 14:213–225, 1998

Winters KC, Bengston P, Dorr D, et al: Prevalence and risk factors of problem gambling among college students. Psychol Addict Behav 12:127–135, 1998

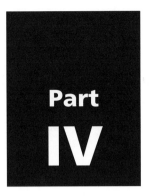

Part

IV

Prevention and Treatment

Chapter 10

Prevention Efforts and the Role of the Clinician

Marc N. Potenza, M.D., Ph.D.
Mark D. Griffiths, Ph.D., C.Psychol.

The importance of prevention efforts in medical practice is profound. Although prevention efforts targeting mental health and addictive disorders are widely used, only limited data are available on their effectiveness. In the area of substance abuse prevention, large-scale structured investigations have been conducted into the effectiveness of individual programs (e.g., Drug Abuse Resistance Education or Project DARE [Clayton et al. 1996]) and annual surveys examining related behaviors (e.g., National Household Drug Abuse Survey [Substance Abuse and Mental Health Services Administration 2003]) have been completed. However, much less work has been done in the prevention realm for problem or pathological gambling. Therefore, although prevention efforts exist for pathological gambling, they are limited in comparison to other areas in the field of mental health and addictive disorders, and their effectiveness at reducing or eliminating problem and pathological gambling among adult populations has not been adequately investigated to date. The aim of this chapter is to review some prevention efforts aimed at problem and pathological gambling in adults and to highlight their relevance for the general psychiatrist. Prevention efforts that target gambling, problem gambling, and pathological gambling among adolescents and teenagers are covered in Chapter 11, "Prevention and Treatment of Adolescent Problem and Pathological Gambling."

Prevention has historically been divided into three stages. The term *primary prevention* has been used to describe measures employed to "prevent the onset of a targeted condition" (U.S. Preventive Services Task Force 1996, p. xli). *Secondary prevention* refers to measures that "identify and treat asymptomatic persons who have already developed risk factors or preclinical disease but in whom the condition is not clinically apparent" (U.S. Preventive Services Task Force 1996, p. xli). *Tertiary prevention* describes efforts targeting individuals with identified disease in which the goals involve restoration of function, including minimizing or preventing disease-related adverse consequences (U.S. Preventive Services Task Force 1996). These divisions of prevention thus focus on different targets, with primary efforts tending to target the general population; secondary efforts, at-risk or vulnerable groups; and tertiary efforts, individuals with an identified disorder.

Given that treatment can be considered a form of tertiary prevention and that behavioral and pharmacological treatments are covered elsewhere in this book (see Chapter 12, "Cognitive and Behavioral Treatments," and Chapter 13, "Pharmacological Treatments"), we focus our discussion of tertiary prevention on "early" efforts, such as gambling help lines (which help guide many individuals who are treatment naïve into treatment settings) and casino self-exclusion practices (which help minimize harm to identified individuals with gambling problems).

Primary Prevention

Primary prevention efforts—often considered the most cost-effective forms of prevention because they help reduce the suffering, cost, and burden associated with a disorder (U.S. Preventive Services Task Force 1996)—include health protection education and counseling. Primary prevention efforts related to problem and pathological gambling have generally involved education initiatives. Examples include television commercials, billboards, bus tails, posters, postcards, and other means of increasing public awareness (Griffiths 2003). Despite their widespread use, most primary prevention efforts aimed at gambling have not been empirically validated. It has been suggested that organizations examine the effectiveness of their interventions—for example, through random telephone surveys (Griffiths 2003). Information concerning the effectiveness of an intervention might include the number of people hearing the advertisement, the extent to which they understand the message, the usefulness or appropriateness of the message, and the extent to which the message prompts behavioral changes (Griffiths 2003).

The content and impact of primary prevention are strongly influenced by knowledge of the effects of the behavior or disorder being targeted. For example, efforts promoting the cessation of smoking tobacco have changed significantly as more information concerning the health impact of tobacco smoke has become available (Slovic 2001). Unfortunately, few large-scale, well-designed studies have been performed to investigate the health impact of different levels or types of gambling (e.g., recreational, problem, and pathological gambling) (National Research Council 1999). Data from existing large-scale surveys are emerging; for example, in the Gambling Impact and Behavior Study, associations were found between problem and pathological gambling and receipt of unemployment benefits and welfare, bankruptcy, arrest, incarceration, poor or fair physical health, and mental health treatment (National Opinion Research Center 1999; Potenza et al. 2001a).

Despite the emergence of data from the Gambling Impact and Behavior Study and other recently published, well-designed, large surveys supporting an association between problem and pathological gambling and adverse measures of functioning (particularly substance use disorders) (Cunningham-Williams et al. 1998; Welte et al. 2001), these investigations have provided little information on either the natural history of gambling behaviors or the nature of the associations. Information from these areas will be very important in conceptualizing gambling within a public health perspective (see Chapter 1, "Gambling and the Public Health") and in generating guidelines for healthy gambling such as those that currently exist for alcohol consumption (Center for Nutrition Policy and Promotion 2000; Dietary Guidelines Advisory Committee 2000; Korn 2000; Korn and Shaffer 1999; Shaffer and Korn 2002).

Although the strongest data exist for an association between adverse measures of health and well-being and problem or pathological levels of gambling, there have been suggestions of adverse health measures in association with less severe gambling in general or within specific gambling venues. For example, a high proportion (83%) of casino-related deaths were found to be sudden cardiac deaths, raising the possibility that, in the authors' words, "gambling activities can be hazardous to one's health, particularly among elderly cardiac patients" (Harvard Medical School Division on Addictions 2000; Jason et al. 1990, p. 116). Direct examination of the relationship between gambling and cardiac health is warranted, particularly because 1) gambling has been shown to lead to sustained increases in cortisol level and blood pressure over several hours of gambling (Meyer et al. 2000); and 2) the use of automated defibrillators in casinos has been reported to be an effective preventive measure in enhancing survival after sudden cardiac arrest (Potenza et al. 2002; Valenzuela et al. 2000).

A separate (but related) general health risk associated with gambling is exposure to tobacco smoke at casinos and other gambling venues. Direct analysis of environmental tobacco smoke in casinos and bingo halls has revealed significant levels of nicotine and mutagens, with measures of airborne mutagenicity correlating highly with nicotine concentrations (Kado et al. 1991). Casino employees have reported secondhand smoke as a health concern (Keith et al. 2001), and casino employees' description of significant exposure to secondhand smoke is supported by the demonstration of postshift increases in serum cotinine levels (Shaffer et al. 1999; Trout et al. 1998). Given the association between gambling and tobacco smoking, particularly problem and pathological gambling and nicotine dependence (Crockford and el-Guebaly 1998; Cunningham-Williams et al. 1998; Petry and Oncken 2002; Potenza et al., in press), exposure to tobacco smoke should be a consideration in the conceptualization of healthy gambling guidelines.

Some primary prevention efforts targeting children and adolescents could influence adult gambling behaviors and thus warrant mentioning. For example, one prevention program involving 289 high school students employed didactic delivery of gambling-related information (Gaboury and Ladouceur 1993). The study showed that the intervention improved students' knowledge, generated a more realistic attitude toward gambling, and resulted in lower gambling severity. A related study demonstrated that among 115 participants chosen at random in a shopping mall, a brochure on gambling provided new information about problem gambling, risky behavior, and the availability of specialized gambling help (Ladouceur et al. 2000b). A third study designed to correct misconceptions and increase knowledge about gambling involved 424 adolescents, used a video format, and found that the intervention had a positive effect in increasing knowledge and in modifying misconceptions toward gambling (Ferland et al. 2002). Despite these promising initial results, it is unclear if positive effects will be maintained into adulthood or if the same interventions employed in adolescent populations would be effective for adults. Research on prevention programs outside the gambling field has suggested that regardless of delivery mode (e.g., didactic lecture, videotapes, posters, pamphlets, guest speakers), the "information only" approach has relatively little effect on behavioral change (Evans and Getz 2003).

Another issue to be considered in primary prevention is the impact of gambling availability on the development of problem and pathological gambling. Gambling has persisted over time in all cultures despite changes in social attitudes and laws permitting or prohibiting gambling (Potenza and Charney 2001). Over the past several decades, the availability of legalized gambling has rapidly increased in the United States and other areas of the world (Potenza et al. 2001a). Data suggest that the increase in availability has been concurrent with increases in the rates of recreational, problem, and pathological gambling (National Opinion Research Center 1999; Shaffer and Hall 2001). For example, a meta-analysis of prevalence estimate studies in North America found higher estimates of problem and pathological gambling in studies performed from 1994 to 1997 than in those from 1977 to 1993 (Shaffer and Hall 2001). The extent to which gambling should be regulated or restricted remains an area of active debate, with the decisions holding considerable potential impact on public health and prevention efforts.

In summary, although primary prevention efforts related to adult gambling exist, they are relatively few, particularly in light of the public health impact of problem and pathological gambling. Moreover, current and future efforts would benefit from empirical validation and additional information on the nature of the mediating factors between gambling and health measures (i.e., potential causality). Such information could lead to guidelines for healthy gambling and more informative and effective public awareness campaigns.

Secondary Prevention

Secondary prevention efforts involve measures that target individuals with risk factors for developing a disorder or with preclinical forms of the disorder. Here we will extend the definition to consider efforts directed toward vulnerable although not necessarily high-risk groups, such as older adults. Secondary prevention measures in general constitute important interventions in general medical settings. For example, brief screening instruments like the CAGE have demonstrated efficacy within general medical settings in facilitating the identification and treatment of individuals with alcohol use problems (Fiellin et al. 2000).

Although it is likely that generalist physicians encounter individuals with gambling problems in their provision of clinical care, the extent to which they are trained to examine for or that they feel comfortable in assessing gambling problems warrants consideration. For example, in a survey of 180 health care providers, 96% reported having knowledge of problem and pathological gambling, but only 30% reported that they inquire about gambling problems when a patient presents with stress-related symptoms (Christensen et al. 2001).

A separate study of directors of health ministries, medical school officials, and experts in the area of substance use and gambling disorders examined office resource needs and cited lack of awareness, knowledge, education, and training in the area of pathological gambling as the most important challenges or barriers confronting physicians (Rowan and Galasso 2000). The authors described a need for enhanced physician training in gambling disorders during all levels of medical training, including through continuing medical education courses.

A significant group of gamblers report health problems as a direct result of their gambling. Possible adverse health consequences of gambling for both the gambler and their partners include depression, insomnia, intestinal disorders, migraines, and other stress-related disorders (Griffiths 2001; Griffiths et al. 1999; Lorenz and Yaffee 1986, 1988). General practitioners routinely ask patients about smoking and drinking, but gambling is generally not discussed (Setness 1997). Mounting evidence suggests that in order to provide optimal care, medical practitioners within all areas—particularly general medical and psychiatric disciplines—require an awareness of the potential impact of gambling on health and well-being and the information and skill necessary to identify and refer or treat individuals affected by problem or pathological gambling. Together, the data suggest that gambling in its most excessive forms should be conceptualized, much like drug addiction, as a significant medical condition (McLellan et al. 2000; Potenza et al. 2001a, 2002).

Efficient screening methods for problem gambling behaviors could be of significant value in general medical settings. Several brief screening instruments for problem and pathological gambling have been developed, and preliminary data suggest that the Early Intervention Gambling Health Test (see Appendix B), an eight-item self-report questionnaire, has high sensitivity and specificity within a primary care setting (Potenza et al. 2002; Sullivan 2000). Although it is too early to develop practice guidelines for problem and pathological gambling prevention efforts within a general medical setting, generalist physicians could regularly assess patients' gambling histories, sensitively broach the topic of the possible existence of gambling problems with patients who are suspected of engaging problematically in gambling, thoughtfully motivate individuals with gambling problems to seek treatment, and appropriately refer individuals with gambling problems to a self-help group such as Gamblers Anonymous (1-800-266-1908 or http://www.gamblersanonymous.org), a local gambling treatment program, or a gambling help line such as that of the National Council on Problem Gambling (1-800-522-4700 or http://www.ncpgambling.org) to facilitate engagement in locally available gambling treatment (Potenza et al. 2002).

Brief screening instruments could also be of significant utility in other settings, including mental health and addiction treatment offices, jails and other forensic facilities, and gambling venues. Individuals within these settings should be aware of the high rates of problem and pathological gambling in specific groups—for example, males, adolescents, and individuals with histories of incarceration or psychiatric (including substance use) disorders. Given the high rates of co-occurrence of gambling and other psychiatric disorders, screening of individuals with problem or pathological gambling for other psychiatric disorders (and vice versa) could enhance tertiary prevention efforts: providing treatment that more effectively reduces the harm associated with each disorder.

Individuals attending gambling venues, particularly pari-mutuel settings, have been found to have high rates of problem and pathological gambling (National Opinion Research Center 1999). As such, they represent important areas for secondary prevention efforts. Toward these ends, many gambling venues train their staff to identify potential problem or pathological gamblers and advertise within the facilities methods for patrons to obtain help (e.g., through gambling help lines or self-exclusion programs, as described below under "Tertiary Prevention").

Specific populations, although at arguably lower risk, might require unique prevention efforts. For example, gambling problems are more prevalent in men than in women, and there are gender-related differences in problem gambling behaviors. For example, women generally begin to gamble and develop problems with gambling later in life, and they more frequently develop problems with nonstrategic, machine-based forms of gambling like casino slot machines (Potenza et al. 2001b; Tavares et al. 2001). As such, prevention efforts for men and women might preferentially target specific venues or age groups. Similarly, older adults are less likely to gamble, to develop gambling-related problems, and to report problems associated with gambling when acknowledging a gambling problem, but they are more likely to engage in and develop problems with specific forms of gambling such as casino slot machines and sweepstakes gambling (Desai et al., in press; Mendez et al. 2000; National Opinion Research Center 1999; Potenza et al., in press). Accordingly, specific secondary prevention efforts for older adults might be needed. These could include screening older adult populations for problem or pathological gambling within extended care facilities or listing problem gambling referral sources in large print on casino slot machines (Potenza et al., in press). Within health care settings, specific groups of older adults might be at increased risk for gambling problems. For example, several case reports have described the emergence or worsening of problem or pathological gambling in individuals being treated with pro-dopaminergic agents for Parkinson's disease (Gschwandtner et al. 2001; Molina et al. 2000; Seedat et al. 2000). Further research is needed to investigate the effectiveness of secondary prevention efforts targeting these and other high-risk or vulnerable populations of adults.

Tertiary Prevention

Tertiary prevention efforts involve reducing disorder-related harm in affected individuals. These efforts, which include behavioral and pharmacological therapies for pathological gambling, are described in Chapters 12 and 13, "Cognitive and Behavioral Treatments," and "Pharmacological Treatments," respectively. Early tertiary prevention efforts involve moving individuals with recently recognized gambling problems into treatment (e.g., through gambling help lines) and using non-treatment-related methods for helping individuals with gambling problems refrain from gambling (e.g., through the availability and maintenance of casino self-exclusion policies).

Gambling help lines are widely used in the United States and elsewhere in the world (Griffiths et al. 1999; Potenza et al. 2000; Sullivan et al. 1994, 1997). For example, the gambling help line operated by the Connecticut Council on Problem Gambling (CCPG) (which predominantly serves Connecticut and two nearby states) routinely receives more than 1,000 telephone calls a year from callers requesting help with gambling problems (Potenza et al. 2000, 2001b); this volume of calls is considerably lower than that experienced by help lines in other states and by the National Council on Problem Gambling help line. In Connecticut, the majority (approximately 85%) of callers reporting a gambling problem say that they have never attended self-help programs or received professional treatment for a gambling problem (Potenza et al. 2000, 2001b). Individuals calling the CCPG help line are routinely referred for self-help and professional treatment, and consequently the gambling help line facilitates the entry of individuals with recently recognized gambling problems into treatment. Given that the toll-free number for the CCPG help line is advertised in general (e.g., on billboards and buses) and prominently at all gambling venues in the state (e.g., at casinos, pari-mutuel locations, and lottery points of purchase and on the backs of lottery tickets), help lines can serve to bridge primary, secondary, and tertiary prevention efforts.

Information from help line callers can help enhance prevention efforts. For example, very few adolescents call the CCPG help line, suggesting that other prevention efforts might be needed to identify adolescents with gambling problems and provide them with appropriate treatment.

Data suggest that other groups (e.g., Hispanic and African American men) are underrepresented in the CCPG help line sample (Potenza et al. 2001b). Differences have been observed in data obtained from help lines serving other geographic regions. For example, a study of data from the gambling help line in the United Kingdom indicates that adolescents use the gambling help line to a greater degree than they do the CCPG help line, and that women use the United Kingdom gambling help line less frequently compared with the CCPG help line (Griffiths et al. 1999; Potenza et al. 2001b). The precise reason for the apparent differences in the findings from the United Kingdom and the United States are not known but could involve differences in subject populations, advertising, or gambling behaviors. For example, adolescents in the United Kingdom more frequently gamble on fruit and slot machines compared with those in the United States, and problems with fruit or slot machine gambling are frequently acknowledged in the United Kingdom and CCPG samples (Griffiths et al. 1999; Potenza et al. 2001b). The extent to which underrepresented populations might be effectively targeted (e.g., through changes in advertising such as the listing of help line contact information in Spanish and English to reach more Hispanic men) requires direct examination. In addition, further work is needed to directly examine the effectiveness of help lines with regard to treatment referral follow-up. That is, information obtained from callers who are willing to be called back several months after initial contact with the help line would be valuable in assessing the extent to which problem gamblers have benefited from the help line intervention.

Self-exclusion policies exist in casinos around the world, including North America. Although the precise rules and regulations vary according to geographic location and individual casino, they generally involve voluntary self-exclusion for a period of time (e.g., 6 months to 5 years) at the risk of being arrested (e.g., for trespassing) if the excludee is found on the premises (Ladouceur et al. 2000a). Little research has been performed on the effectiveness of casino self-exclusion practices. The only research article examining the effectiveness of a casino self-exclusion program involved 220 self-selected individuals (Ladouceur et al. 2000a). Respondents were predominantly male, middle-aged, and married, and the majority (95%) were pathological gamblers according to their South Oaks Gambling Screen scores (Ladouceur et al. 2000a). Although the majority (97%) reported believing they would refrain from casino gambling during the self-exclusion period, reports from prior excludees (24% of the sample) suggested otherwise (Ladouceur et al. 2000a). Specifically, 36% of the prior excludees reported engaging in casino gambling during their prior exclusion period (Ladouceur et al. 2000a). However,

30% of the prior excludees reported complete gambling abstinence during the prior exclusion period (Ladouceur et al. 2000a). Future research is needed to define factors predictive of success in casino self-exclusion programs and to enhance effective enforcement of the agreements.

Conclusion

Prevention efforts aimed at reducing or eliminating adult problem and pathological gambling are at a relatively early stage of development. Increased knowledge regarding the impact of different types and levels of gambling behaviors on health and well-being would be extremely valuable in generating guidelines for healthy gambling and primary prevention efforts. An increased understanding of high-risk and vulnerable populations—facilitated through biological, psychological/psychiatric, and social investigations—and the natural histories of gambling behaviors within these groups will help enhance secondary and early tertiary prevention efforts. As in other fields of medicine, the effectiveness of individual prevention strategies will need to be empirically validated. Targeted efforts in these areas should lead to a decrease in suffering attributable to problem and pathological gambling.

References

Center for Nutrition Policy and Promotion: Dietary Guidelines for Americans, 5th Edition. Washington, DC, U.S. Department of Agriculture, 2000. Available at: http://www.usda.gov/cnpp/dietary_guidelines.html. Accessed December 20, 2003.

Christensen MH, Patsdaughter CA, Babington LM: Health care providers' experiences with problem gamblers. J Gambl Stud 17:71–79, 2001

Clayton RR, Cattarello AM, Johnstone BM: The effectiveness of Drug Abuse Resistance Education (Project DARE): 5-year follow-up results. Prev Med 25:307–318, 1996

Crockford DN, el-Guebaly N: Psychiatric comorbidity in pathological gambling: a critical review. Can J Psychiatry 43:43–50, 1998

Cunningham-Williams RM, Cottler LB, Compton WM III, et al: Taking chances: problem gamblers and mental health disorders—results from the St. Louis Epidemiologic Catchment Area Study. Am J Public Health 88:1093–1096, 1998

Desai RA, Maciejewski PK, Dausey DJ, et al: Health correlates of recreational gambling in older adults. Am J Psychiatry (in press)

Dietary Guidelines Advisory Committee: Discussion of proposed changes, in Report of the Dietary Guidelines Advisory Committee on Dietary Guidelines for Americans, 2000. Washington, DC, U.S. Department of Agriculture, Agricultural Research Service, 2000, pp 20–61. Available at: http://www.ars.usda.gov/dgac. Accessed December 20, 2003.

Evans RI, Getz J: Social inoculation, in Encyclopedia of Primary Prevention and Health Promotion. Edited by Gullotta TP, Bloom M. New York, Kluwer Academic, 2003, pp 1028–1033

Ferland F, Ladouceur R, Vitaro F: Prevention of problem gambling: modifying misconceptions and increasing knowledge. J Gambl Stud 18:19–29, 2002

Fiellin DA, Reid MC, O'Connor PG: Screening for alcohol problems in primary care: a systematic review. Arch Intern Med 160:1977–1989, 2000

Gaboury A, Ladouceur R: Evaluation of a prevention program for pathological gambling among adolescents. J Prim Prev 14:21–28, 1993

Griffiths MD: Gambling—an emerging area of concern for health psychologists. J Health Psychol 6:477–479, 2001

Griffiths MD: Raising gambling awareness through advertising. GamCare News 16:14–15, 2003

Griffiths MD, Scarfe A, Bellringer P: The UK national telephone gambling help-line—results on the first year of operation. J Gambl Stud 15:83–90, 1999

Gschwandtner U, Aston J, Renaud S, et al: Pathologic gambling in patients with Parkinson's disease. Clin Neuropharmacol 24:170–172, 2001

Harvard Medical School Division on Addictions: Gambling mortality. The WAGER 5(41):1–3, 2000. Available at: http://www.thewager.org/backissues.htm. Accessed December 19, 2003.

Jason DR, Taff ML, Boglioli LR: Casino-related deaths in Atlantic City, New Jersey 1982–1986. Am J Forensic Med Pathol 11:112–123, 1990

Kado NY, McCurdy SA, Tesluk SJ, et al: Measuring personal exposure to airborne mutagens and nicotine in environmental tobacco smoke. Mutat Res 261:75–82, 1991

Keith MM, Cann B, Brophy JT, et al: Identifying and prioritizing gaming workers' health and safety concerns using mapping for data collection. Am J Ind Med 39:42–51, 2001

Korn DA: Expansion of gambling in Canada: implications for health and social policy. CMAJ 163:61–64, 2000

Korn DA, Shaffer HJ: Gambling and the health of the public: adopting a public health perspective. J Gambl Stud 15:289–365, 1999

Ladouceur R, Jacques C, Giroux I, et al: Analysis of a casino's self-exclusion policy. J Gambl Stud 16:453–460, 2000a

Ladouceur R, Vezina L, Jacques C, et al: Does a brochure about pathological gambling provide new information? J Gambl Stud 16:103–108, 2000b

Lorenz VC, Yaffee RA: Pathological gambling: psychosomatic, emotional and marital difficulties reported by the gambler. Journal of Gambling Behavior 2:40–45, 1986

Lorenz VC, Yaffee RA: Pathological gambling: psychosomatic, emotional and marital difficulties as reported by the spouse. Journal of Gambling Behavior 4:13–26, 1988

McLellan AT, Lewis DC, O'Brien CP, et al: Drug dependence, a chronic medical illness. JAMA 284:1689–1695, 2000

Mendez MF, Bronstein YL, Christine DL: Excessive sweepstakes participation by persons with dementia. J Am Geriatr Soc 48:855–856, 2000

Meyer G, Hauffa BP, Schedlowski M, et al: Casino gambling increases heart rate and salivary cortisol in regular gamblers. Biol Psychiatry 48:948–953, 2000

Molina JA, Sainz-Artiga MJ, Fraile A, et al: Pathologic gambling in Parkinson's disease: a behavioral manifestation of pharmacologic treatment? Mov Disord 15:869–872, 2000

National Opinion Research Center: Gambling Impact and Behavior Study: Report to the National Gambling Impact Study Commission. Chicago, IL, National Opinion Research Center at the University of Chicago, 1999. Available at: http://www.norc.uchicago.edu/new/gamb-fin.htm. Accessed December 13, 2003.

National Research Council: Pathological Gambling: A Critical Review. Washington, DC, National Academy Press, 1999

Petry NM, Oncken C: Cigarette smoking is associated with increased severity of gambling problems in treatment-seeking gamblers. Addiction 97:745–753, 2002

Potenza MN, Charney DS: Pathological gambling: a current perspective. Semin Clin Neuropsychiatry 6:153–154, 2001

Potenza MN, Steinberg MA, McLaughlin SD, et al: Illegal behaviors in problem gambling: analysis of data from a gambling helpline. J Am Acad Psychiatry Law 28:389–403, 2000

Potenza MN, Kosten TR, Rounsaville BJ: Pathological gambling. JAMA 286:141–144, 2001a

Potenza MN, Steinberg MA, McLaughlin SD, et al: Gender-related differences in the characteristics of problem gamblers using a gambling helpline. Am J Psychiatry 158:1500–1505, 2001b

Potenza MN, Fiellin DA, Heninger GR, et al: Gambling: an addictive behavior with health and primary care implications. J Gen Intern Med 17:721–732, 2002

Potenza MN, Steinberg MA, McLaughlin SD, et al: Characteristics of tobacco-using problem gamblers calling a gambling helpline. Am J Addict, in press

Rowan MS, Galasso CS: Identifying office resource needs to help prevent, assess and treat patients with substance use and pathological gambling disorders. J Addict Dis 19:43–58, 2000

Seedat S, Kesler S, Niehaus DJH, et al: Pathological gambling behaviour: emergence secondary to treatment of Parkinson's disease with dopaminergic agents. Depress Anxiety 11:185–186, 2000

Setness PA: Pathological gambling: when do social issues become medical issues? (editorial). Postgrad Med 102:13–18, 1997

Shaffer HJ, Hall MN: Updating and refining prevalence estimates of disordered gambling behaviour in the United States and Canada. Can J Public Health 92:168–172, 2001

Shaffer HJ, Korn DA: Gambling and related mental disorders: a public health analysis. Annu Rev Public Health 23:171–212, 2002

Shaffer HJ, Vander Bilt J, Hall MN: Gambling, drinking, smoking and other health risk activities among casino employees. Am J Ind Med 36:365–378, 1999

Slovic P: Smoking: Risk, Perception and Policy. Thousand Oaks, CA, Sage, 2001

Substance Abuse and Mental Health Services Administration: 2002 National Survey on Drug Use and Health. Rockville, MD, Substance Abuse and Mental Health Services Administration, Office of Applied Studies, 2003. Available at: http://www.samhsa.gov/oas/nhsda.htm. Accessed January 1, 2003.

Sullivan SG: Pathological gambling in New Zealand: the role of the GP. New Ethicals Journal 3:11–18, 2000

Sullivan SG, Abbott M, McAvoy B, et al: Pathological gamblers—will they use a new telephone hotline? N Z Med J 107:313–315, 1994

Sullivan SG, McCormick R, Sellman JD: Increased requests for help by problem gamblers: data from a gambling crisis telephone hotline. N Z Med J 110:380–383, 1997

Tavares H, Zilberman ML, Beites FJ, et al: Gender differences in gambling progression. J Gambl Stud 17:151–159, 2001

Trout D, Decker J, Mueller C, et al: Exposure of casino employees to environmental tobacco smoke. J Occup Environ Med 40:270–276, 1998

U.S. Preventive Services Task Force: Guide to Clinical Preventive Services, 2nd Edition. Baltimore, MD, Williams & Wilkins, 1996

Valenzuela TD, Roe DJ, Nichol G, et al: Outcomes of rapid defibrillation by security officers after cardiac arrest in casinos. N Engl J Med 343:1206–1209, 2000

Welte J, Barnes G, Wieczorek W, et al: Alcohol and gambling pathology among U.S. adults: prevalence, demographic patterns and comorbidity. J Stud Alcohol 62:706–712, 2001

Prevention and Treatment of Adolescent Problem and Pathological Gambling

Jeffrey L. Derevensky, Ph.D.
Rina Gupta, Ph.D.
Laurie Dickson, M.A.

The past decade has witnessed a renewed interest in the negative aspects associated with gambling. National commissions in Australia, New Zealand, the United Kingdom, and the United States have begun to examine the economic benefits and social costs of the expansion of gambling. Simultaneously, researchers have begun to assess the negative consequences of problem and pathological gambling for high-risk populations. Although problem and pathological gambling have been viewed as primarily affecting adults, recent evidence indicates that gambling is a popular youth activity. It is estimated that between 4% and 8% of adolescents currently have a serious gambling problem and that another 10%–14% of adolescents remain at risk for developing a serious gambling problem (Jacobs 2000; National Research Council 1999; Shaffer and Hall 1996) (see Chapter 5, "Adolescents and Young Adults").

Given the growing number of gambling opportunities, the attractiveness of many of those opportunities to youths, and the widespread proliferation of easily accessible gambling venues, a greater need for scientifically based prevention and treatment programs has become apparent. Efforts to understand the economic, social, and psychological costs of problem gambling have increased in recent years. The recognition that adolescents are particularly susceptible to developing risk-related problem behaviors in general (Baer et al. 1998; Jessor 1998; Luthar et al. 2000) and gambling-related problems in particular (Gupta and Derevensky 1998a; National Research Council 1999; Wynne et al. 1996) amplifies the necessity for effective prevention initiatives targeting adolescents.

Prevention Initiatives

Structured studies that investigate the prevention of adolescent pathological and problem gambling, as well as the translation of study findings into science-based prevention initiatives, have been particularly scarce (Dickson et al. 2002). A new conceptual approach, *prevention science*, has more recently formed the basis of school-based prevention efforts (Coie et al. 1993). If prevention initiatives are to be effective, they must be conceptually driven from adolescent research on resiliency, given that gambling remains a highly socially acceptable adult activity (Azmier 2000) and an activity that is frequently engaged in by adolescents (Jacobs 2000).

The resiliency literature is predicated on findings that some individuals appear to be more immune to adversity, deprivation, and stress than others. Although it remains inevitable that all individuals face stressful life events, children and adolescents have different adaptive behaviors and often unique ways of coping. Resiliency is believed to be related to biological self-righting dispositions in human development (Waddington 1957) and to the protective mechanisms that work in the presence of stressors (Rutter 1987; Werner and Smith 1982). As such, resilient youths are able to cope more effectively with stressful situations and emotional distress in ways that enable them to develop appropriate adaptive behaviors.

If gambling prevention programs are to incorporate the promotion of resiliency among youths as their overarching goal, a positive profile includes the development of 1) effective problem-solving skills, including the ability to think abstractly and the ability to generate and implement solutions to cognitive and social problems; 2) social competence, encompassing flexibility, effective communication skills, empathy for others, and prosocial behavior; 3) autonomy, self-efficacy, and self-control; and 4) a sense of purpose, success orientation, motivation, and optimism (Brown et al. 2001).

Although prevention programs aimed at minimizing gambling problems are relatively new, efforts aimed at preventing the use of tobacco, alcohol, and drugs among youths have existed for many years. Current prevention efforts in the fields of alcohol and drug abuse have focused on the concepts of risk and protective factors and their interaction (Brounstein et al. 1999). Such efforts seek to prevent or limit the effects of risk factors (variables associated with a high probability of onset, greater severity, and longer duration of major mental health problems) and increase protective factors (conditions that improve an individual's resistance to risk factors and disorders). As such, prevention efforts are designed to enhance resiliency. Successful risk-focused prevention programs need to focus on eliminating, reducing, or minimizing risk factors associated with negative outcomes, whether they are associated with problematic levels of gambling or alcohol or drug use. Evidence of resiliency in children (e.g., Garmezy 1985; Rutter 1987; Werner 1986) has expanded the prevention field from a risk prevention framework to one that includes both risk-prevention and the fostering of protective factors. Protective factors have been shown to moderate or buffer the effects of individual vulnerabilities or environmental adversity such that the adaptational trajectory becomes more positive than if the protective factors were not at work (Masten et al. 1990).

Risk and protective factors that operate on the level of the individual include physiological factors (e.g., biochemical and genetic), personality variables, values and attitudes, early and persistent problem behaviors, and substance use. These risk and protective factors operate in the family domain through family management practices, parental modeling, familial structure (e.g., two-parent vs. single-parent homes), and family climate (including conflict resolution and socioemotional parent–child bonding). The peer domain is also particularly relevant in the prevention of adolescent risk behaviors because risk and protective factors have been found to operate through peer associations, social expectancies with regard to substance use, and school performance. The school context also affects an adolescent's attitudes and behavior. Academic performance, school bonding (perceived connectedness with school), and school policies have been found either to buffer risk factors for substance abuse or to be precursors of unsuccessful coping and the development of substance abuse. At the community level, risk and protective factors affect adolescent risk behavior via accessibility to substances. At the broadest level of societal environment, laws and attitude norms, including those portrayed in the media, influence adolescent risk behaviors.

In an attempt to conceptualize the current state of knowledge concerning the risk factors associated with problem gambling, Dickson et al.

(2002) used a similar paradigm based on the current knowledge of youths with severe gambling problems. The following were included: 1) individual domain factors—including poor impulse control, high sensation seeking, unconventionality, poor psychological functioning, low self-esteem, early and persistent problem behaviors, and early initiation; 2) familial domain factors—including familial history of substance abuse, parental attitudes, and modeling of deviant behavior; 3) peer domain factors—including social expectancies and reinforcement by peers; and 4) societal domain factors—including school difficulties, access to the substance or problem activity, and societal norms.

Although some research has been undertaken to identify risk factors for adolescent problem gambling (Derevensky and Gupta 2000; Dickson et al. 2002; Griffiths and Wood 2000; Gupta and Derevensky 2000), no published studies to date have directly investigated protective mechanisms—or, more generally, resiliency—with respect to youth problem gambling. Protective factors that have been examined across other youthful addictions can be grouped into three general categories: care and support, dispositional attributes (such as positive and high expectations), and opportunities for participation (Werner 1989). These characteristics encompass each domain that fosters resiliency in youths.

Research on adolescent alcohol and substance abuse suggests that no single approach to prevention will be uniformly successful (Baer et al. 1998). A combination of strategies that nurture resilience in youths appears to be most effective. Such a multimodal approach may be most effective in the prevention of youth gambling problems and other high-risk behaviors. This kind of approach requires scientific validation before it will achieve widespread implementation. The validation process should include data on information dissemination; prevention education (the development of critical life skills, social skills, and effective coping skills); nongambling activities; problem gambling identification and referral; community-based processes (training community members and agencies in prevention); and active lobbying for social policies that aim to reduce risk factors and enhance protective factors.

Successful prevention programs adapt their prevention materials and strategies to the developmental levels of the target audience. Coping strategies and social, academic, and economic pressures change with age (Eisenberg et al. 1997). Evaluation measures should be congruent with developmental differences associated with age-related coping and adaptive behaviors. Incorporating current information regarding the profiles of problem gamblers and knowledge acquired from research on risk prevention models should help to shape future curriculum efforts more effectively.

Treatment for Adolescents

Although several treatment modalities appear promising for adults (see Chapter 12, "Cognitive and Behavioral Treatments," and Chapter 13, "Pharmacological Treatments"), the efficacy of treatment programs for youths with gambling problems has been largely untested. Psychodynamic techniques have reportedly been successfully used in the treatment of an adolescent male with a severe gambling problem (Harris 1964). More recently, Ladouceur and his colleagues argued for a cognitive-behavioral approach to treating both adults and youths with gambling problems (e.g., Bujold et al. 1994; Ladouceur and Walker 1996, 1998; Ladouceur et al. 1994, 1998).

In one of the few empirically based treatment studies, four male adolescents with pathological gambling underwent cognitive-behavioral therapy (Ladouceur et al. 1994). Cognitive therapy incorporating five elements (information about gambling, cognitive interventions, problem-solving training, relapse prevention, and social skills training) was individually provided for a period of approximately 3 months (averaging 17 sessions). The results suggested clinically significant improvement concerning the perception of control when gambling and a significant reduction in severity of gambling problems. One month after termination of treatment, one adolescent had relapsed. At assessments 3 and 6 months after treatment, the remaining three adolescents had sustained therapeutic treatment gains and were abstinent, with none of the adolescents meeting DSM criteria for pathological gambling at the last follow-up assessment. The treatment duration necessary for adolescents with pathological gambling was relatively short compared with that required for adults. These findings should be interpreted cautiously given the small sample.

Compared with other adolescents, adolescents with problem and pathological gambling have been found to exhibit evidence of abnormal physiological resting states and to display greater emotional distress, more depressive symptoms, poor coping and adaptive behaviors, low self-esteem, higher excitability, and higher rates of comorbidity with other addictive behaviors.

Adolescent problem gamblers also frequently present with a host of interpersonal, emotional, academic, behavioral, and familial problems, with gambling being used as an unsuccessful solution to these underlying troubles. Many patients exhibit clinical depression and symptoms of attention-deficit/hyperactivity disorder.

Money is not always the predominant underlying reason for gambling among adolescents (Gupta and Derevensky 1998a, 1998b). Rather, money is merely used as a means to enable youths to continue gambling.

Through their gambling, adolescents frequently dissociate and escape into another world, often with altered egos and repression of unpleasant daily events or long-term problems (Gupta and Derevensky 2000). Adolescents with serious gambling problems report that all their problems disappear while they are gambling. They report that betting on the outcome of a sporting event, watching the spinning reels of a video lottery terminal machine or an electronic gaming machine, or scratching an instant lottery ticket provides a rush, increasing their heart rate and intensifying excitement. These same physiological responses are often recalled whether the individual is winning or losing (the near-miss phenomenon).

For most youths with gambling problems, a good day is when their money lasts all day. In contrast, a bad day is when their money is quickly lost. Once all money is lost, their preexisting problems (e.g., financial, parental, familial, academic, legal, vocational, peer, interpersonal, and social) reappear, with additional gambling-related problems only compounding existing problems. A 19-year-old male provided this metaphor: "My life is like a tree, with one branch being a thief, another being a liar, and another being out of school and work. If you cut off a branch, you haven't gotten to the root of my problem…gambling." Yet underlying this individual's gambling problems were a number of psychological problems. Gambling became his outlet, a way of enhancing his self-esteem (when he gambled large sums of money) and a way to "kill time."

Reasons for gambling parallel those of adults. Adolescents report gambling for entertainment and excitement and as a way to win money easily (generally so that they can continue gambling or pay gambling debts), and to enhance their self-esteem. They report that nothing parallels the excitement they receive from gambling "when they are winning or when they are losing."

An Example of an Adolescent Treatment Program

Gupta and Derevensky (2000) reported general success from their treatment program for adolescents with gambling problems. Their therapeutic approach not only addresses the severity of the individual's gambling problem and the concomitant negative problems associated with the gambling behavior (e.g., loss of trust, disrupted familial relationships, lost friends, and economic indebtedness) but also seeks to identify and treat any underlying psychological problems.

In the Gupta and Derevensky (2000) study, individual therapy was conducted weekly, with daily sessions provided when required (the total number of sessions therefore ranged between 20 and 50). Therapy included a detailed intake interview and assessment, the individual's acceptance of a gambling problem, identification and addressing of key personal problems, development of effective coping skills and adaptive behavior, restructuring of free time, involvement of familial and social supports, cognitive restructuring of erroneous beliefs, establishment of debt repayment schedules, and relapse prevention (a more detailed explanation can be found in the study). Antidepressant medications were also commonly used in conjunction with traditional psychotherapy.

Essential to success of treatment programs are the development and enhancement of effective coping strategies. Empirical data and clinical observations of adolescents with severe gambling problems reveal that they are more likely to engage in gambling behavior when they are bored or under stress; these adolescents also use gambling as a means to socialize with their peers. Finding alternative strategies is both individualistic and important in the recovery process.

Further study is needed to examine the potential of specific pharmacotherapies in the treatment of pathological gambling among adolescents. Several antidepressants (e.g., fluvoxamine and paroxetine) have also been shown in placebo-controlled trials to be effective in the short-term treatment of pathological gambling in adults independent of depressive symptoms (see Chapter 13, "Pharmacological Treatments").

Assessing Outcome of Treatment

Outcome measures used for success include abstinence for 6 months, a healthy lifestyle (e.g., improved socialization with nongambling friends, a return to or improvement in school or work), improved peer and family relationships, and no marked signs of depressive symptoms, delinquent behavior, or excessive use of alcohol or drugs. Adolescents are generally followed up for 2 years after treatment. Although no matched sample control group was used in the initial studies, and analyses of long-term (multiyear) follow-ups have yet to be undertaken, the results of the study seem promising.

Little is known about the short-term and long-term treatment effects for adolescents with serious gambling problems. Few clinicians specialize in providing treatment for youths with gambling problems, and those who are trained report that very few adolescents present themselves for treatment (Derevensky et al. 2003). Nevertheless, considerable empirical data on the prevalence rates of gambling problems in youths demonstrate the need for prevention initiatives and outreach programs.

Conclusion

The development of prevention initiatives and their acceptance into school-based curriculums should be conceptualized into a wider picture of problem and risk-taking behaviors among youths (Dickson et al. 2002). For those providing treatment, approaches need to be broad, targeting issues beyond gambling. Gambling problems among youths are generally a reflection of deeper underlying social, emotional, and behavioral difficulties.

Problem gambling during adolescence remains a growing social problem with serious psychological, sociological, and economic implications. Although the incidence of severe gambling problems among youths remains relatively small, the pervasiveness of the problem and the long-term, devastating consequences to those individuals, their families, and their friends are enormous. A general lack of public and parental awareness that severe gambling problems exist among youths—and that adolescents perceive themselves as invulnerable—raises serious mental health, public health, and social policy concerns.

Social policies concerning problem gambling among youths are relatively scarce. Although most states and provinces have established statutes delineating the legal minimum age of entry to casinos, most have yet to establish legislative policies with regard to adolescent gambling. Laws designed to prohibit underage gambling should be seriously enforced, and subsequent prevention and treatment programs for adolescent gambling need to be comprehensive, taking into account developmental, social, and psychological factors.

References

Azmier JJ: Canadian Gambling Behavior and Attitudes: Summary Report (CWF Publ No 200001). Calgary, AB, Canada West Foundation, 2000

Baer JS, MacLean MG, Marlatt GA: Linking etiology and treatment for adolescent substance abuse: toward a better match, in New Perspectives on Adolescent Risk Behavior. Edited by Jessor R. New York, Cambridge University Press, 1998, pp 182–220

Brounstein PJ, Zweig JM, Gardner SE: Understanding Substance Abuse Prevention: Toward the 21st Century: A Primer on Effective Programs. Rockville, MD, Substance Abuse and Mental Health Services Administration, Center for Substance Abuse Prevention, Division of Knowledge Development and Evaluation, 1999

Brown JH, D'Emidio-Caston M, Benard B: Resilience Education. Thousand Oaks, CA, Corwin Press, 2001

Bujold A, Ladouceur R, Sylvain C, et al: Treatment of pathological gamblers: an experimental study. J Behav Ther Exp Psychiatry 25:275–282, 1994

Coie J, Watt N, West S, et al: The science of prevention. Am Psychol 48:1013–1022, 1993

Derevensky JL, Gupta R: Youth gambling: a clinical and research perspective. eGambling (2):1–10, 2000. Available at: http://www.camh.net/egambling/issue2/feature. Accessed December 22, 2003.

Derevensky JL, Gupta RA, Winters K: Prevalence rates of youth gambling problems: are the current rates inflated? J Gambl Stud 19:405–425, 2003

Dickson LM, Derevensky JL, Gupta R: The prevention of gambling problems in youth: a conceptual framework. J Gambl Stud 18:97–159, 2002

Eisenberg N, Fabes R, Guthrie I: Coping with stress in roles of regulation and development, in Handbook of Children's Coping: Linking Theory and Intervention (Issues in Clinical Child Psychology Series). Edited by Wolchik SA, Sandler IN. New York, Plenum, 1997, pp 41–70

Garmezy N: The NIMH-Israeli high-risk study: commendations, comments, and cautions. Schizophr Bull 11:349–353, 1985

Griffiths M, Wood RT: Risk factors in adolescence: the case of gambling, video-game playing, and the internet. J Gambl Stud 16:199–225, 2000

Gupta R, Derevensky JL: Adolescent gambling behavior: a prevalence study and examination of the correlates associated with problem gambling. J Gambl Stud 14:319–345, 1998a

Gupta R, Derevensky JL: An empirical examination of Jacob's General Theory of Addictions: do adolescent gamblers fit the theory? J Gambl Stud 14:17–49, 1998b

Gupta R, Derevensky JL: Adolescents with gambling problems: from research to treatment. J Gambl Stud 16:315–342, 2000

Harris HI: Gambling addiction in an adolescent male. Psychoanal Q 33:513–525, 1964

Jacobs DF: Juvenile gambling in North America: an analysis of long term trends and future prospects. J Gambl Stud 16:119–152, 2000

Jessor R: New perspectives on adolescent risk behavior, in New Perspectives on Adolescent Risk Behavior. Edited by Jessor R. New York, Cambridge University Press, 1998, pp 1–12

Ladouceur R, Walker M: A cognitive perspective on gambling, in Trends in Cognitive and Behavioural Therapies. Edited by Salkovskis PM. New York, Wiley, 1996, pp 89–120

Ladouceur R, Walker M: The cognitive approach to understanding and treating pathological gambling, in Comprehensive Clinical Psychology. Edited by Bellack AS, Hersen M. New York, Pergamon, 1998, pp 588–601

Ladouceur R, Boisvert JM, Dumont J: Cognitive-behavioral treatment for adolescent pathological gamblers. Behav Modif 18:230–242, 1994

Ladouceur R, Sylvain C, Letarte H, et al: Cognitive treatment of pathological gamblers. Behav Res Ther 36:1111–1119, 1998

Luthar SS, Cicchetti D, Becker B: The construct of resilience: a critical evaluation and guidelines for future work. Child Dev 71:543–562, 2000

Masten A, Best K, Garmezy N: Resilience and development: contributions from the study of children who overcome adversity. Dev Psychopathol 2:425–444, 1990

National Research Council: Pathological Gambling: A Critical Review. Washington, DC, National Academy Press, 1999

Rutter M: Psychosocial resilience and protective mechanisms. Am J Orthopsychiatry 57:316–331, 1987

Shaffer HJ, Hall MN: Estimating the prevalence of adolescent gambling disorders: a quantitative synthesis and guide toward standard gambling nomenclature. J Gambl Stud 12:193–214, 1996

Waddington CH: The Strategy of Genes. London, Allen & Unwin, 1957

Werner EE: Resilient offspring of alcoholics: a longitudinal study from birth to age 18. J Stud Alcohol 47:34–40, 1986

Werner EE: High risk children in young adulthood: a longitudinal study from birth to 32 years. Am J Orthopsychiatry 59:72–81, 1989

Werner EE, Smith RS: Vulnerable but Invincible: A Study of Resilient Children. New York, McGraw-Hill, 1982

Wynne HJ, Smith GJ, Jacobs DF: Adolescent Gambling and Problem Gambling in Alberta. Report prepared for the Alberta Alcohol and Drug Abuse Commission. Edmonton, AB, Canada, Wynne Resources, 1996

Chapter

12

Cognitive and Behavioral Treatments

David C. Hodgins, Ph.D.
Nancy M. Petry, Ph.D.

General-population surveys consistently reveal that almost 40% of individuals with pathological gambling in their lifetime do not meet the criteria for pathological gambling in the past year (Hodgins et al. 1999). This finding suggests that a significant proportion of pathological gamblers have recovered or are "in recovery." A variety of routes can lead to recovery. These routes include formal treatments specifically focused on gambling cessation, such as residential programs, outpatient groups, and individual counseling. In addition or alternatively, individuals can obtain treatment for other mental health concerns in which gambling behaviors are addressed indirectly. Gamblers Anonymous, which capitalizes on peer support, has also become widely available. The most frequently traveled pathway may in fact be no treatment at all: self-recovery (Hodgins et al. 1999).

Regardless of the recovery pathway that an individual chooses to travel, similar change strategies may be used (Hodgins and el-Guebaly 2000). From open-ended descriptions provided by recovered gamblers, both treated and nontreated, we derived a categorization scheme. The majority of these strategies fall under the rubric of cognitive-behavioral mechanisms, and many are the focus of cognitive-behavioral interventions.

Types of Cognitive-Behavioral Therapies

Treatment approaches vary in their relative focus on cognitive versus cognitive and behavioral change techniques. In the cognitive approach, gambling is seen as arising from the individual's beliefs and attitudes about control, luck, prediction, and chance (Ladouceur and Walker 1996; Toneatto 2002). The goal of therapy is to identify and change cognitive distortions that are maintaining gambling. In more broad-based cognitive-behavioral approaches, gambling is thought to be maintained by both cognitive and behavioral factors, with treatment utilizing both types of techniques.

These broad-based cognitive-behavioral approaches are typically designed as individual or group-based multi-session therapies. Another trend within the gambling treatment area is to offer brief interventions, applied in a self-directed workbook format (Blaszczynski 1998; Hodgins and Makarchuk 2002) or as one-session interventions (Robson et al. 2002).

Earlier treatments for gambling problems included aversion and desensitization techniques (e.g., Barker and Miller 1966; Koller 1972). Gamblers Anonymous incorporates a number of cognitive and behavioral strategies that can be used alone or with other approaches, as well as specific behavioral strategies such as self-exclusion policies (Nowatzki and Williams 2002) and financial management (National Council on Problem Gambling 2000).

Cognitive Therapy Approaches

Rationale for Cognitive Therapy Approaches

Observational studies in which gamblers verbalize their cognitions reveal that more than 70% of gambling-related thoughts are illogical (Gaboury and Ladouceur 1989; Griffiths 1994; Ladouceur and Dubé 1997). A fundamental cognitive error of gamblers is the *illusion of control*, the perception that one can influence the outcome of a randomly determined event. For example, casino gamblers engage in *strategies* to predict or cause the roulette numbers or dice outcomes. In experimental situations, participants place a higher monetary value on lottery tickets that they have chosen in comparison to tickets that have been assigned to them (Langer 1983). They also wager more money when they "control" a game of roulette by being the one who throws the ball (Ladouceur and Mayrand 1987).

Although much of the research has been conducted with social gamblers, Toneatto (2002) described the types of distortions found in pathological gamblers. The distortions of pathological gamblers include illusions of control such as overinterpretation of cues (a bodily feeling that a win is imminent); magnification of gambling skill (feeling that one is a better slot player because of experience); superstitious behavior (wearing special clothes); control over luck; illusory correlation (environmental signs that a win is likely); attributional biases (a streak of losses signals a win); selective memory (of wins vs. losses); and probability biases (incorrect beliefs of randomness).

Cognitive Therapy Techniques

Cognitive therapy comprises four major components: education, increasing awareness about cognitive errors, raising doubt about the validity of irrational cognitions, and cognitive restructuring. In terms of education, many gamblers lack awareness about the random nature of gambling. Therapists can instruct or remind them that each outcome is independent regardless of whether they appear linked. For example, dice do not "remember" that they have not produced double sixes in a few rolls—each roll is independent. Slot machines work from random number generators, so the time since the last win is not meaningful in predicting future wins. Continuing to play because one is "due to win" is not a productive strategy.

Basic information about gambling may increase patients' awareness of how specific cognitive errors influence their personal gambling. Socratic-type questions are then used: What kind of gambling do the patients prefer? How do they decide when to gamble (e.g., lucky streaks or signs)? How do they explain their wins or losses? When they have a losing streak, do they believe that they are more likely to win in the near future? (Toneatto 2002).

In addition to Socratic questioning to uncover cognitive errors, the patient can self-monitor cognitions associated with gambling. Office-based exercises can also elicit these cognitions in vivo. The patient can verbalize cognitions during the activities, which are audiotaped and examined in detail (Griffiths 1994; Ladouceur and Walker 1996).

The next component of cognitive therapy is to have the patient challenge the validity of cognitions. What is accurate and inaccurate about each thought or belief? What rational statement could replace each irrational one? For example, can the patient really predict when he or she will win? Some patients are easily convinced that their cognitions are flawed. Others will need to collect experiential evidence to disconfirm their belief. The goal of the therapist is to maintain an interested and collaborative stance and to use Socratic-type questioning to help patients begin to doubt their cognitions.

The final component of therapy is to teach patients to challenge their cognitions in vivo when faced with urges to gamble. The patient is asked between sessions to self-monitor gambling or strong gambling urges or cravings. The standard thought record from cognitive therapy is used, including a description of situational, emotional, and cognitive precipitants; sequences of events leading to gambling; and challenges to any irrational cognitions. This component of therapy is typically the largest of the four and continues until the patient begins to internalize some of the ideas and techniques.

Cognitive Therapy Outcome Data

Earlier uncontrolled case reports suggested that treatment focusing on modifications of cognitions could lead to cessation or reduction of gambling (Bujold et al. 1994; Ladouceur et al. 1998; Sylvain and Ladouceur 1992; Toneatto and Sobell 1990; Walker 1992). More recently, Ladouceur and his colleagues completed two randomized trials. In the first (Sylvain et al. 1997), individual therapy was compared with a control condition in which participants waited several months before initiating treatment. Treated participants reported less gambling and increased perceived self-control over gambling at 12 months, compared with those on the waiting list. However, the treatment intervention did not represent a pure cognitive therapy intervention. It included four components; in addition to cognitive therapy, participants received problem-solving training, social skills training, and relapse prevention. In a subsequent trial (Ladouceur et al. 2001), a purer form of cognitive therapy was assessed in a similar research design. The intervention included cognitive therapy plus relapse prevention, which also focused on dealing with cognitive distortions associated with situations that were of high risk for relapse. After 3 months, the treated group had better outcomes than the waiting-list group, and gains were maintained up to 12 months in the treated group.

Although these two randomized trials represent an improvement in methodology compared with previous reports, intention-to-treat analyses were not conducted. Only participants who completed treatment, 63% in the first study and 53% in the second, were included in the outcome evaluation. The generalizability of the results is limited by lack of knowledge about the outcomes of those who dropped out of the study.

Cognitive-Behavioral Approaches

Rationale for Cognitive-Behavioral Approaches

Whereas the cognitive model focuses on cognitions, other models are more broadly based. Sharpe and Tarrier (1993; Sharpe 2002) provided an integrative model describing the maintenance of problem gambling by both cognitive and behavioral factors. According to this model, stimuli that become associated with gambling over time can develop into triggers for gambling. These stimuli can be external (situations, times, places) or internal (affect, cognitions). Once a trigger is encountered, it leads to an involuntary response of heightened autonomic arousal that is accompanied by gambling-related cognitions (e.g., "I feel lucky today") and urges to gamble. Whether or not a person gambles is mediated by coping skills. Treatment involves interventions that target coping skill deficits such as the inability to control autonomic arousal, poor problem-solving skills, inability to delay reinforcement, and poor ability to challenge cognitions.

Cognitive-Behavioral Techniques

A basic technique of cognitive-behavioral therapies is the functional analysis. It consists of identifying triggers or precipitants to gambling. Certain events, days, times, people, and emotions have been paired with gambling in the past and may precipitate gambling episodes or urges. Common triggers include available cash; free or unstructured time (weekends, days off); arguments or interpersonal problems; and boredom, anger, or depression. Gambling episodes are broken into triggers and are then evaluated for both positive and negative consequences. For example, after having an argument with his or her spouse over financial concerns, a gambler may head straight to the casino. The positive effects of gambling may include the possibility of winning and avoiding the spouse. The negative effects of gambling would include losing more money. These negative effects lead to more arguments or to the trigger itself, thereby creating a vicious cycle—gambling to avoid arguments, and gambling leading to more arguments.

Other aspects of cognitive-behavioral therapy include increasing reinforcement derived from nongambling sources to compete with the reinforcers associated with gambling. Patients can be provided with a "leisure checklist" that contains lists of activities and hobbies. They can check ones that they once liked to do, or ones that they might consider trying. Activities that are inexpensive or free are represented, as well as solo and social activities. The gambler is encouraged to try activities in the upcoming week, with the theory that the development of other reinforcing activities may compete with the reinforcement derived from the problem behavior and hence reduce the probability of gambling. Specifically, rewarding activities (going to the movies, gardening, or playing golf) should be planned for high-risk times (e.g., weekends or payday). Precommitment strategies are utilized, such as telephoning an old friend while in the therapist's office to set a date and time to meet for coffee to increase the probability that a healthier behavior will occur.

In other sessions, gamblers are taught to brainstorm for new ways of managing both expected and unexpected triggers and to handle cravings and urges to gamble. They may also be taught other behavioral techniques such as assertiveness training or relaxation training. These cognitive-behavioral strategies can be delivered either alone or in conjunction with cognitive therapy, such as the therapy described above that addresses more specifically the erroneous cognitions associated with gambling (see "Cognitive Therapy Techniques").

Outcome Data for Cognitive-Behavioral Therapy

Case studies of successful reductions in gambling after cognitive-behavioral therapy have been noted in several reports (Arribas and Martinez 1991; Bannister 1977; Sharpe and Tarrier 1992). Results of one randomized trial from Spain are available (Echeburua et al. 1996). Gamblers were randomized to one of four conditions: 1) individual stimulus control and in vivo exposure with response prevention, 2) group cognitive restructuring, 3) a combination of the first two treatments, or 4) a waiting-list control condition. At 6 months, treatments 1 and 2 performed better than the combined or control groups. At 12 months, rates of abstinence or minimal gambling were higher in the individual-treatment group (69%) compared with the group cognitive restructuring (38%) and combined-treatment (38%) groups. Thus, the combination of group cognitive therapy and individual stimulus control and exposure appeared to diminish the effectiveness of either intervention delivered alone.

These same investigators reported on the effectiveness of providing relapse prevention as a follow-up to their 6-week individual intervention (Echeburua et al. 2000, 2001). Treatment completers were randomly assigned to no further treatment or relapse-prevention therapy delivered in either group or individual format. The relapse-prevention intervention involved training participants to identify and cope with relapse precipitants, including social pressure, negative affect, and interpersonal conflict. Over a 12-month follow-up period, 86% of the individual and 78% of the group intervention participants did not relapse, compared with 52% of the group who received no further treatment.

In summary, controlled outcome data support the effectiveness of a cognitive-behavioral intervention that includes stimulus control and response prevention, as well as cognitive therapy combined with problem solving, social skills training, and relapse prevention (Sylvain et al. 1997). N.M. Petry (unpublished data, 1998) developed an eight-session manualized cognitive-behavioral treatment for pathological gamblers. It includes the cognitive-behavioral strategies described above (in "Cognitive-Behavioral Techniques") and also devotes one session to modifying erroneous cognitions. A group of 220 pathological gamblers have been enrolled in a study evaluating the efficacy of this approach. The cognitive-behavioral therapy is either delivered by a professionally trained counselor or completed alone by the patient in a self-help workbook. Both conditions are compared with referral to Gamblers Anonymous. Preliminary data suggest that the professionally delivered therapy has greater efficacy relative to the workbook or the Gamblers Anonymous referral.

Brief Interventions

Rationale for Brief Interventions

One challenge for treatment providers is attracting individuals to treatment programs; studies show that fewer than 8% of pathological gamblers receive treatment (National Gambling Impact Study Commission 1999; Productivity Commission 1999). Individuals with earlier stage or less severe problems, those who are concerned about privacy and convenience, and those who want to handle the problem on their own are less likely to attend treatment (Hodgins and el-Guebaly 2000). To these individuals, workbooks may be an attractive, accessible, and cost-effective alternative to formal treatment programs or self-help groups. Self-directed workbooks have been used in a number of areas of behavior change such as phobias, depression, headaches, smoking, and exercise. Unlike Petry's study discussed above, meta-analyses of comparisons between self-help interventions and no-treatment control conditions or therapist-directed interventions indicate that self-help approaches are more effective than control conditions and are as effective as the same programs administered by therapists (Gould and Clum 1993). Similarly, brief face-to-face treatments have been developed for alcohol use disorders (Burke et al. 2003), and these brief treatments have the largest and most consistently positive empirical database of the large array of alcohol treatments (Miller et al. 2003).

Brief Treatment Outcome

Dickerson et al. (1990) randomly assigned 29 gamblers to complete a workbook alone or in conjunction with a single in-depth interview. The workbook included cognitive-behavioral and motivational enhancement techniques to reduce ambivalence regarding change. Both groups reported significant reductions in gambling at a 6-month follow-up. Hodgins et al. (2001) used media advertising to recruit 102 problem gamblers into a larger study. The subjects were randomly assigned to receive a workbook only, to receive a workbook plus a telephone motivational enhancement intervention, or to be placed on a waiting list. At the 1-month follow-up, a significant advantage was found for the telephone intervention and workbook condition. Compared with the workbook-only group, those who received the motivational intervention and workbook reduced gambling throughout a 2-year follow-up period (Hodgins et al. 2001; Hodgins et al., in press a). These results support the use of media to recruit participants who are reluctant to seek formal treatment. Further research is needed to better understand the types of gamblers who are best helped by these brief treatments.

Three additional trials of brief treatment approaches are in progress. Hodgins has been conducting a trial that focuses on providing relapse prevention in the form of information pamphlets to pathological gamblers who have quit gambling but who are not attending support groups ($N=168$). In another ongoing trial being conducted by Hodgins, concerned family members and friends of pathological gamblers ($N=185$) are receiving self-directed materials to help them better cope with the situation and to help get the gambler to seek treatment. Finally, Petry has been evaluating three brief treatments for problem gamblers ($N=150$): 5 minutes of brief advice about reducing gambling, a one-session motivational intervention, and a four-session intervention that combines motivational interviewing and cognitive-behavioral therapy. All these trials include a long-term follow-up evaluation.

Behavioral Aversion and Desensitization Approaches

Rationale for Behavioral Aversion and Desensitization

In early models, pathological gambling was considered to result from a combination of classical and operant conditioning, whereby gambling is reinforced through intermittent schedules of reinforcement (Petry 2002). Reinforcers can be financial but also include arousal, excitement, and negative reinforcers such as escape from aversive states (Diskin and Hodgins 1999).

Behavioral Aversion and Desensitization Outcome

Earlier behavioral therapies focused on aversion techniques to decrease positive reinforcement and increase negative reinforcement associated with gambling. Typically, this therapy involved applying electrical shocks to gamblers as they gambled, won at gambling, or thought about the positive effects associated with gambling. The use of aversion therapy in treating pathological gamblers is described in case reports (e.g., Barker and Miller 1966; Koller 1972). Although some of these reports indicated beneficial effects, few patients were treated, and limited follow-up periods were included.

Throughout the 1970s, the use of broader behavioral therapies emerged. Behavioral monitoring, covert sensitization, relaxation techniques, and spousal contingency contracting were provided alone or in conjunction with aversion therapy (National Research Council 1999). Beneficial effects were noted in the bulk of the published case reports (but see Greenberg and Marks 1982; Kraft 1970), but the samples were often small, the durations of follow-up periods were limited, and attrition rates were high (Greenberg and Rankin 1982). More recently, other techniques have been used in conjunction with cognitive and cognitive-behavioral therapy. In imaginal desensitization, patents are taught relaxation skills to reduce physical tension and are then instructed to imagine experiencing and resisting a series of cues to gambling. With in vivo exposure, the gambler approaches the actual gambling environment, often in a series of steps graded by difficulty, and practices coping skills while not gambling. Blaszczynski (1998) provided a detailed description of these techniques.

In one study, McConaghy et al. (1983) compared aversion therapy and imaginal desensitization in a randomized design and found that both groups improved. Each group, however, consisted of only 10 gamblers, which limited the ability to uncover differences between the treatments. In another study using a larger sample, 120 pathological gamblers were randomly assigned to one of four inpatient treatments: aversion therapy, imaginal desensitization, in vivo desensitization, or imaginal relaxation. Participants receiving imaginal desensitization reported better outcomes at 1 month and up to 9 years later, although only about half the sample was successfully followed up (McConaghy et al. 1991). More research is needed to isolate the independent or unique contributions of these behavioral techniques alone or in conjunction with other cognitive and cognitive-behavioral treatments for gambling.

Gamblers Anonymous

Gamblers Anonymous is one of the most popular interventions for pathological gamblers. Although it is not theoretically based, Gamblers Anonymous utilizes a number of behavioral techniques. First, members provide one another with positive reinforcement for refraining from gambling. Members state their duration of abstinence at each meeting, and special rewards are provided for abstinence anniversaries, such as pins, certificates, or special meetings. Second, Gamblers Anonymous provides an alternative social activity to compete with gambling itself. Sponsors and call lists are utilized so that a gambler can telephone another member and receive social support and encouragement 24 hours a day, 7 days a week. Finally, the notion of taking one day at a time encourages the gambler to make behavioral decisions on truncated time frames, within which self-controlled decisions may be more likely (see Petry 2001).

Although over 1,000 Gamblers Anonymous chapters exist in North America alone, little published literature exists on its efficacy. Researchers who have done observational work concur that most Gamblers Anonymous attendees do not become actively involved in the fellowship (Preston and Smith 1985; Rosecrance 1988; Taber and Chaplin 1988; Turner and Saunders 1990). In a review of the number of meetings attended by new participants, Stewart and Brown (1988) found that of 232 attendees only 7.5% obtained a 1-year abstinence pin. Almost one-quarter of new attendees never came back for a second meeting, and almost three-quarters attended 10 or fewer meetings.

Some data suggest that the effectiveness of Gamblers Anonymous can be enhanced by participation in professional treatment programs. Russo et al. (1984) evaluated 124 patients who completed a Veterans Administration program that combined individual and group psychotherapy with Gamblers Anonymous attendance. Of the 60 patients who completed the follow-up evaluation, 33 (55%) reported abstinence. Attendance at Gamblers Anonymous meetings and engagement in professional therapy were each associated with long-term abstinence. Taber et al. (1987) reported on 6-month outcomes of admissions to the same facility. Abstinence was reported by 56% of the patients, and again Gamblers Anonymous attendance was associated with abstinence. Lesieur and Blume (1991) contacted 72 of 119 gamblers who had attended an inpatient program that combined professional and 12-step treatment for gambling and substance use disorders. Although engagement in Gamblers Anonymous was not assessed, 46 patients (64%) reported abstinence from gambling 6–14 months after completing treatment. Although a sizable proportion of gamblers who received professional treatment and attended Gamblers Anonymous meetings maintained abstinence, the professional treatment was provided in an inpatient setting, and the vast majority of the gamblers were male.

Stinchfield and Winters (1996) reported on the outcomes of 1,342 patients entering outpatient treatment in Minnesota. Of the full sample, almost half became actively engaged in professional treatment, and about one-third attended one or more Gamblers Anonymous meetings. Those who completed treatment demonstrated reductions in gambling and psychosocial problems, but Gamblers Anonymous attendance was not a significant predictor of outcomes in that study.

More recently, Petry (2003) evaluated Gamblers Anonymous participation rates in Connecticut among 342 consecutive admissions to professional treatment programs for gambling. More than half the patients had attended Gamblers Anonymous prior to initiating professional treatment for their gambling. Of those gamblers with a history of Gamblers Anonymous attendance, 41% came to five or more professional treatment sessions in a 2-month period—compared with only 24% of treatment seekers who did not attend Gamblers Anonymous meetings. Moreover, Gamblers Anonymous attendees in the professional treatment sessions had a higher rate of gambling abstinence (48% vs. 36%). The number of Gamblers Anonymous meetings attended was significantly and independently associated with abstinence. Although these results suggest potential effectiveness of Gamblers Anonymous when combined with professional therapy, the data do not demonstrate the efficacy of Gamblers Anonymous in reducing gambling, because random assignment procedures were not used. These outcome data simply suggest that gamblers who choose to attend Gamblers Anonymous (and receive professional treatment) do better than those who present for professional treatment but do not become actively engaged in either treatment modality.

Other Focused Approaches

Self-Exclusion

In some jurisdictions, local government or casino policy allows individuals to voluntarily ban themselves from gambling venues such as casinos and racetracks. Typically, the exclusion is for a defined time period lasting from 3–12 months to a lifetime. The person may be excluded from one facility or from all facilities in the jurisdiction. When an individual enrolls in the program, his or her photograph is circulated to the security officers of the facilities. The individual is also typically provided with information about local treatment resources. Sanctions for being caught on the premises can range from a formal request to leave to fines or legal charges of trespassing. Winnings are sometimes confiscated.

A review of self-exclusion programs concluded that participants are typically male and have gambling problems and significant financial debts (Nowatzki and Williams 2002). However, evidence is limited on the effectiveness of such programs. The only known evaluation (Ladouceur et al. 2000) focused on a small group of gamblers who were seeking their second exclusion from a Quebec casino. In this group, 64% had not entered the casino during their first exclusion (6 or 12 months), and 30% had stopped gambling. Those who had violated the ban did so a median of six times. Only 10% had sought treatment. In summary, more research is required to understand the role that exclusion policies can have in helping pathological gamblers overcome their problems.

Financial Counseling

Financial counseling is often included in cognitive-behavioral programs as an adjunctive service, with the rationale that financial pressures are a common trigger for gambling. The service is often offered on an individual basis, but self-directed materials are also available (National Council on Problem Gambling 2000). Gamblers Anonymous offers "pressure relief" sessions, which assist in providing advice for managing large debts. Other options include referral to consumer credit organizations or bankruptcy lawyers. Typically, Gamblers Anonymous and gambling therapists recommend that the gambler relinquish all control of finances to a spouse or another person. The use of such strategies as an adjunct to psychotherapy may be an important area of research.

Unresolved Issues in Cognitive-Behavioral Treatment

The ability to treat pathological gamblers continues to increase, although there are limited empirical data on issues related to effectiveness (Oakley-Browne et al. 2000). In Table 12–1, the small number of randomized clinical trials published to date are summarized. A number of ongoing trials will provide valuable insights, but other issues remain. These include abstinence versus control as a treatment goal, the impact of comorbid disorders, and the relative efficacy of group versus individual treatment.

Abstinence Versus Control as a Treatment Goal

The optimal treatment goal continues to be debated. The Gamblers Anonymous model requires abstinence from all types of gambling; for example, a slot machine gambler must cease buying lottery tickets. The rationale for total abstinence is that another form of gambling can either become problematic or act as a precipitant to relapse to another form. Most treatment providers and outcome study protocols (e.g., Sylvain et al. 1997) also recommend abstinence.

Table 12–1. Published randomized trials of cognitive and behavioral treatments

Study	Sample	Design	Findings
Dickerson et al. 1990	Media-recruited problem gamblers—Australia	Workbook vs. workbook and assessment interview	Both groups improved over 6 months
Echeburua et al. 1996	Outpatient pathological gamblers—Spain	Individual stimulus control and in vivo exposure vs. group cognitive restructuring vs. combined vs. waiting-list control group	Individual condition had better outcomes than group or combined over 6 months
Echeburua et al. 2000, 2001	Outpatient pathological gamblers after treatment—Spain	Relapse prevention group vs. individual relapse prevention vs. no treatment	Both treatments superior to no treatment over 12 months
Hodgins et al. 2001	Media-recruited problem gamblers—Canada	Telephone motivational enhancement vs. workbook vs. waiting-list control group	Motivational enhancement superior over 12 months
Ladouceur et al. 2001	Outpatient pathological gamblers—Canada	Cognitive therapy vs. waiting list	Treatment superior to waiting list at 3 months; improvement maintained over 12 months
McConaghy et al. 1983	Inpatient pathological gamblers—Australia	Aversion therapy vs. imaginal desensitization	Improvement in both groups over 12 months
McConaghy et al. 1991	Inpatient pathological gamblers—Australia	Aversion therapy vs. imaginal desensitization vs. in vivo desensitization vs. imaginal relaxation	Imaginal desensitization group showed most improvement over 1 month and 9 years
Sylvain et al. 1997	Outpatient pathological gamblers—Canada	Individual cognitive-behavioral therapy vs. waiting list	Treatment superior to waiting list over 12 months

However, other models allow the client to set a personal outcome goal that can include reduced or "controlled" gambling. Strict abstinence goals may discourage gamblers from seeking treatment, and flexibility may open the doors to more treatment seekers. In the alcohol field, alcoholic individuals who begin treatment with a controlled drinking goal often move toward an abstinence goal (Hodgins et al. 1997).

The controlled gambling option is supported by follow-up data on a small group of treated pathological gamblers (63 of 120; Blaszczynski et al. 1991). When interviewed 2–9 years after treatment, 18 (29%) were abstinent, 20 (32%) continued to gamble in an uncontrolled fashion, and 25 (40%) were "controlled gamblers." The controlled gamblers resembled the abstinent gamblers in terms of other indicators of psychosocial stability. These data are based on the small group of gamblers who were successfully followed up (52%), so the data need to be interpreted with caution. Clinical trials comparing treatments with varying treatment goals are necessary.

Treatment of Comorbidity

Pathological gambling co-occurs with a number of psychiatric disorders. The strongest association is with substance abuse disorders, with 25%–63% of gamblers reporting substance use disorders (Crockford and el-Guebaly 1998; Petry and Pietrzak, in press). Mood disorders—including depression, bipolar disorder, and anxiety disorders—are also common. Evidence is mixed for other comorbidities such as attention-deficit disorder, eating disorders, and schizophrenia and other psychotic disorders (Crockford and el-Guebaly 1998).

It is unclear how the various comorbid disorders are related to pathological gambling. A variety of models are possible, and different models may apply to different pathological gamblers. In some cases, for example, depression may be precipitated by the psychosocial consequences of a gambling problem. Alternatively, gambling may reflect a maladaptive attempt to self-medicate depressive symptoms. Alcohol is typically served in gambling venues, which might increase the likelihood that a heavy drinker would be exposed to gambling. Individuals recovering from alcoholism may also turn to gambling as an alternative way to shift their emotional state.

The impact that comorbid disorders have on outcome requires further study. In one prospective study, pathological gamblers with a history of clinical depression had poorer gambling outcomes, whereas those who battled a concurrent substance abuse problem had more success (Hodgins et al., in press b). It is also unclear what the best management approaches are for comorbid disorders. One possibility with cognitive-behavioral approaches is to expand the focus to include the comorbid disorder. Cognitive-behavioral treatments have been validated for substance use and depression in particular. Alternatively, pharmacological approaches to the comorbid disorders can be combined with psychosocial treatments.

Relative Efficacy of Group Versus Individual Treatment

An interesting disconnection between treatment outcome literature and clinical practice is that empirical validation efforts focus almost exclusively on individually based models, whereas clinical service is most frequently offered in a group format. In the only study that compared individual therapy with combined group and individual therapy, an advantage for individual therapy alone was found (Echeburua et al. 1996). However, the group and individual therapies were different (cognitive group therapy and in vivo response prevention individual therapy), making the results difficult to interpret.

Group-based treatments have some benefits over individual therapy (Coman et al. 2002), including the enhancement of social skills, the opportunity to learn and practice new behaviors in advance of trying them outside the group, and the opportunity to get feedback and support from other group members. In short, the patients can learn from the struggles and successes of other members as well as from their own. On the other hand, gamblers may be more reluctant to attend group therapy than individual therapy. Confidentiality concerns, whether imagined or actual, may also be a barrier. Therapeutic groups operate in a very different fashion than Gamblers Anonymous, which some patients may find troublesome. Finally, those who drop out will affect not only themselves but also other patients in the group.

Conclusion

Much more research on cognitive and cognitive-behavioral therapies is needed. New studies should isolate unique techniques that may be independently associated with beneficial response and the processes by which patients change. These studies should also consider the impact of specific aspects of treatment—such as financial counseling, self-exclusion programs, controlled gambling, comorbidity, and format—in improving outcomes. Although no one treatment is likely to benefit all patients, the availability of a number of empirically validated treatments may attract more gamblers into treatment and may contribute to helping more gamblers begin the recovery process on their own.

References

Arribas MP, Martinez JJ: Individual treatment of pathologic gamblers: case descriptions (in Spanish). Analisis y Modificacion de Conducta 17:255–269, 1991

Bannister G: Cognitive and behavior therapy in a case of compulsive gambling. Cognit Ther Res 1:223–227, 1977

Barker JC, Miller M: Aversion therapy for compulsive gambling. Lancet 1:491–492, 1966

Blaszczynski A: Overcoming Compulsive Gambling: A Self-Help Guide Using Cognitive Behavioral Techniques. London, Robinson, 1998

Blaszczynski A, McConaghy N, Frankova A: Control versus abstinence in the treatment of pathological gambling: a two to nine year follow-up. Br J Addict 86:299–306, 1991

Bujold A, Ladouceur R, Sylvain C, et al: Treatment of pathological gamblers: an experimental study. J Behav Ther Exp Psychiatry 25:275–282, 1994

Burke BL, Arkowitz H, Menchola M: The efficacy of motivational interviewing: a meta-analysis of controlled clinical trials. J Cons Clin Psychol 71:843–861, 2003

Coman GJ, Evans BJ, Burrows GD: Group counselling for problem gambling. Br J Guid Counc 30:145–158, 2002

Crockford DN, el-Guebaly N: Psychiatric comorbidity in pathological gambling: a critical review. Can J Psychiatry 43:43–50, 1998

Dickerson M, Hinchy J, Legg England S: Minimal treatments and problem gamblers: a preliminary investigation. J Gambl Stud 6:87–102, 1990

Diskin KM, Hodgins DC: Narrowing of attention and dissociation in pathological video lottery gamblers. J Gambl Stud 15:17–28, 1999

Echeburua E, Baez C, Fernandez-Montalvo J: Comparative effectiveness of three therapeutic modalities in psychological treatment of pathological gambling: long term outcome. Behavioural and Cognitive Psychotherapy 24:51–72, 1996

Echeburua E, Fernandez-Montalvo J, Baez C: Relapse prevention in the treatment of slot-machine pathological gambling: long-term outcome. Behav Ther 31:351–364, 2000

Echeburua E, Fernandez-Montalvo J, Baez C: Predictors of therapeutic failure in slot-machine pathological gamblers following behavioural treatment. Behavioural and Cognitive Psychotherapy 29:379–383, 2001

Gaboury A, Ladouceur R: Erroneous perceptions and gambling. J Soc Behav Pers 4:411–420, 1989

Gould RA, Clum GA: A meta-analysis of self-help treatment approaches. Clin Psychol Rev 13:169–186, 1993

Greenberg D, Marks I: Behavioural psychotherapy of uncommon referrals. Br J Psychiatry 141:148–153, 1982

Greenberg D, Rankin H: Compulsive gamblers in treatment. Br J Psychiatry 140:364–366, 1982

Griffiths MD: The role of cognitive bias and skill in fruit machine gambling. Br J Psychol 85:351–369, 1994

Hodgins DC, el-Guebaly N: Natural and treatment-assisted recovery from gambling problems: comparison of resolved and active gamblers. Addiction 95:777–789, 2000

Hodgins DC, Makarchuk K: Becoming a Winner: Defeating Problem Gambling: A Self-Help Manual for Problem Gamblers. Calgary Addiction Centre, Calgary Regional Health Authority, 2002

Hodgins DC, Leigh G, Milne R, et al: Drinking goal selection in behavioral self-management treatment of chronic alcoholics. Addict Behav 22:247–255, 1997

Hodgins DC, Wynne H, Makarchuk K: Pathways to recovery from gambling problems: a general population survey. J Gambl Stud 15:93–104, 1999

Hodgins DC, Currie SR, el-Guebaly N: Motivational enhancement and self-help treatments for problem gambling. J Consult Clin Psychol 69:50–57, 2001

Hodgins DC, Currie SR, el-Guebaly N, et al: Brief motivational treatment for pathological gambling: a 24-month follow-up. Psychol Addict Behav (in press a)

Hodgins DC, Peden N, Cassidy E: The association between comorbidity and outcome in pathological gambling: a prospective follow-up of recent quitters. J Gambl Stud (in press b)

Koller KM: Treatment of poker-machine addicts by aversion therapy. Med J Aust 1:742–745, 1972

Kraft T: A short note on forty patients treated by systematic desensitization. Behav Res Ther 8:219–220, 1970

Ladouceur R, Dubé D: Erroneous perceptions in generating random sequences: identification and strength of a basic misconception in gambling behavior. Swiss Journal of Psychology 56:256–259, 1997

Ladouceur R, Mayrand M: The level of involvement and the timing of betting in roulette. J Psychol 121:169–176, 1987

Ladouceur R, Walker M: A cognitive perspective on gambling, in Trends in Cognitive and Behavioural Therapies. Edited by Salkovskis PM. New York, Wiley, 1996, pp 89–120

Ladouceur R, Sylvain C, Letarte H, et al: Cognitive treatment of pathological gamblers. Behav Res Ther 36:1111–1119, 1998

Ladouceur R, Jacques C, Giroux I, et al: Analysis of a casino's self-exclusion program. J Gambl Stud 16:453–460, 2000

Ladouceur R, Sylvain C, Boutin C, et al: Cognitive treatment of pathological gambling. J Nerv Ment Dis 189:774–780, 2001

Langer EJ: The Psychology of Control. Beverly Hills, CA, Sage, 1983

Lesieur HR, Blume SB: Evaluation of patients treated for pathological gambling in a combined alcohol, substance abuse and pathological gambling treatment unit using the Addiction Severity Index. Br J Addict 86:1017–1028, 1991

McConaghy N, Armstrong MS, Blaszczynski A, et al: Controlled comparison of aversive therapy and imaginal desensitization in compulsive gambling. Br J Psychiatry 142:366–372, 1983

McConaghy N, Blaszczynski A, Frankova A: Comparison of imaginal desensitisation with other behavioural treatments of pathological gambling: a two- to nine-year follow-up. Br J Psychiatry 159:390–393, 1991

Miller WR, Wilbourne PL, Hettema JE: What works? a summary of alcohol treatment outcome research, in Handbook of Alcoholism Treatment Approaches: Effective Alternatives, 3rd Edition. Edited by Hester R, Miller WR. Boston, MA, Allyn & Bacon, 2003, pp 13–63

National Council on Problem Gambling and National Endowment for Financial Education: Personal Financial Strategies for the Loved Ones of Problem Gamblers. Greenwood Village, CO, National Endowment for Financial Education, 2000

National Gambling Impact Study Commission: National Gambling Impact Study Commission Final Report. Washington, DC, National Gambling Impact Study Commission, 1999

National Research Council: Pathological Gambling: A Critical Review. Washington, DC, National Academy Press, 1999

Nowatzki NR, Williams RJ: Casino self-exclusion programmes: a review of the issues. International Gambling Studies 2:3–25, 2002

Oakley-Browne MA, Adams P, Mobberley PM: Interventions for pathological gambling. Cochrane Database Syst Rev (2):CD001521, 2000

Petry NM: Pathological gamblers, with and without substance use disorders, discount delayed rewards at high rates. J Abnorm Psychol 110:482–487, 2001

Petry NM: Psychosocial treatments for pathological gambling: current status and future directions. Psychiatr Ann 32:192–196, 2002

Petry NM: Patterns and correlates of Gamblers Anonymous attendance in pathological gamblers seeking professional treatment. Addict Behav 28:1049–1062, 2003

Petry NM, Pietrzak RH: Comorbidity of substance use and gambling disorders, in Dual Diagnosis and Treatment: Substance Abuse and Comorbid Disorders, 2nd Edition. Edited by Kranzler HR, Tinsley J. New York, Marcel Dekker, in press

Preston FW, Smith RW: Delabeling and relabeling in Gamblers Anonymous: problems with transferring the Alcoholics Anonymous paradigm. Journal of Gambling Behavior 1:97–105, 1985

Productivity Commission: Australia's Gambling Industries (Report No 10). Canberra, AusInfo, 1999

Robson E, Edwards J, Smith G, et al: Gambling decisions: an early intervention program for problem gamblers. J Gambl Stud 18:235–255, 2002

Rosecrance J: Active gamblers as peer counselors. Int J Addict 23:751–766, 1988

Russo AM, Taber JI, McCormick RA, et al: An outcome study of an inpatient treatment program for pathological gamblers. Hosp Community Psychiatry 35:823–827, 1984

Sharpe L: A reformulated cognitive-behavioral model of problem gambling: a biopsychosocial perspective. Clin Psychol Rev 22:1–25, 2002

Sharpe L, Tarrier N: A cognitive-behavioural treatment approach for problem gambling. Journal of Cognitive Psychotherapy 6:193–203, 1992

Sharpe L, Tarrier N: Towards a cognitive-behavioural theory of problem gambling. Br J Psychiatry 162:407–412, 1993

Stewart RM, Brown RIF: An outcome study of Gamblers Anonymous. Br J Psychiatry 152:284–288, 1988

Stinchfield R, Winters K: Effectiveness of Six State-Supported Compulsive Gambling Treatment Programs in Minnesota. Minneapolis, Compulsive Gambling Program, Mental Health Division, Minnesota Department of Human Services, 1996

Sylvain C, Ladouceur R: Correction cognitive et habitudes de jeu chez les joueurs de poker video. Can J Behav Sci 24:479–489, 1992

Sylvain C, Ladouceur R, Boisvert JM: Cognitive and behavioral treatment of pathological gambling: a controlled study. J Consult Clin Psychol 65:727–732, 1997

Taber JI, Chaplin MP: Group psychotherapy with pathological gamblers. Journal of Gambling Behavior 4:183–196, 1988

Taber JI, McCormick RA, Ramirez LR: The prevalence and impact of major stressors among pathological gamblers. Am J Psychiatry 146:1618–1619, 1987

Toneatto T: Cognitive therapy for problem gambling. Cognitive and Behavioral Practice 9:191–199, 2002

Toneatto T, Sobell LC: Pathological gambling treated with cognitive behavior therapy: a case report. Addict Behav 15:497–501, 1990

Turner DN, Saunders D: Medical relabeling in Gamblers Anonymous: the construction of an ideal member. Small Group Research 21:59–78, 1990

Walker M: The Psychology of Gambling (International Series in Experimental Social Psychology). New York, Pergamon, 1992

Pharmacological Treatments

Eric Hollander, M.D.
Alicia Kaplan, M.D.
Stefano Pallanti, M.D.

Despite an association between pathological gambling and measures of adverse functioning, little is widely known regarding effective treatments, particularly pharmacotherapies, for pathological gambling. In this chapter we summarize current pharmacological treatment strategies for pathological gambling and the rationales for their use.

Several core psychopathological domains within pathological gambling could conceivably be targeted for treatment: 1) impulsive symptoms (arousal); 2) compulsive symptoms (anxiety reduction); and 3) addictive symptoms (symptoms of withdrawal). Although pathological gambling is classified as an impulse control disorder, it has also been described as an obsessive-compulsive spectrum disorder within the impulsive cluster (Hollander 1993). The urges, pleasure seeking, and reduction in judgment capability (unrealistic evaluation of one's own abilities) seen in pathological gamblers resemble similar characteristics seen in individuals with bipolar disorder. These features—along with high rates of psychiatric comorbidity with bipolar spectrum and other mood disorders, substance abuse and dependence, and attention-deficit/hyperactivity disorder (ADHD)—help provide neuropsychopharmacological frameworks for treatment (see Chapter 4, "Categorization").

Neurobiological investigations have shown evidence of involvement by the serotonergic (Blanco et al. 1996; DeCaria et al. 1996, 1998; Moreno et al. 1991), noradrenergic (DeCaria et al. 1998; Roy et al. 1988), and dopaminergic systems (Bergh et al. 1997; Comings 1998; Perez de Castro et al. 1997) in the etiology of pathological gambling (see Chapter 9, "Biological Basis for Pathological Gambling"). Pharmacological treatments that manipulate these neurotransmitter systems, as well as the γ-aminobutyric acid (GABA) system (Johannessen 2000), have shown potentially promising results in the early stages of understanding and treating pathological gambling.

Currently, no existing medications have been approved by the U.S. Food and Drug Administration for the treatment of pathological gambling. In this chapter we focus on the results of double-blind, placebo-controlled studies (Table 13–1) because of the high placebo response rates in drug treatment trials for pathological gambling. Disorders that commonly co-occur with pathological gambling—such as substance abuse and dependence disorders, bipolar disorder, major depressive disorder, and ADHD—influence choices in the use of pharmacotherapeutic agents, because treatment should ultimately target all symptom domains in the individual patient.

Serotonin Reuptake Inhibitors

Serotonin reuptake inhibitors, which are first-line treatments for obsessive-compulsive disorder (Hollander and Pallanti 2002), have shown efficacy for obsessive-compulsive spectrum disorders such as body dysmorphic disorder (Hollander et al. 1999; Phillips et al. 2002). It appears that serotonin reuptake inhibitors have both anticompulsive and anti-impulsive effects, although there seems to be a longer therapeutic lag time in the compulsively driven disorders (Hollander 1998). Further support for the use of serotonin reuptake inhibitors in treating pathological gambling arises from evidence of serotonergic dysfunction (Blanco et al. 1996; DeCaria et al. 1996, 1998; Moreno et al. 1991) and the pharmacological treatment studies described below.

Fluvoxamine

Three studies have examined the effectiveness of fluvoxamine in treating pathological gambling. In a pilot study by Hollander et al. (1998), 10 patients with pathological gambling completed an 8-week single-blind

Table 13–1. Double-blind, placebo-controlled trials in pathological gambling

Drug (trade name)	Study reference	Design/ duration	Sample size	Daily dosage range	Mean daily dose (± SD)	Outcome
SSRIs						
Fluvoxamine (Luvox)	Hollander et al. 2000b	Crossover 16 weeks (8 weeks each active/placebo), 1-week placebo lead-in	15 enrolled, 10 completers	100–250 mg	195 mg (±50)	Of 10 completers, 7 were responders according to the PG-CGI and PG-YBOCS; fluvoxamine was superior to placebo, particularly at end of 16 weeks.
Fluvoxamine (Luvox)	Blanco et al. 2002	Parallel design, 6 months	32 enrolled, 13 completers (3 fluvoxamine and 10 placebo)	200 mg	200 mg	Fluvoxamine was not statistically significant from placebo in overall sample except in males and young patients.
Paroxetine (Paxil)	Kim et al. 2002	Parallel design, 8 weeks, 1-week placebo lead-in	53 enrolled, 41 completers (20 paroxetine and 21 placebo)	20–60 mg	51.7 mg (±13.1)	Paroxetine group significantly improved compared with placebo group according to CGI.
Paroxetine (Paxil)	Grant et al. 2003	Parallel design, 16-week trial	76 enrolled, 45 completers (21 paroxetine and 24 placebo)	10–60 mg	50 mg (±8.3)	Paroxetine and placebo groups showed comparable improvement; placebo response rate was high.

Table 13–1.   Double-blind, placebo-controlled trials in pathological gambling (*continued*)

Drug (trade name)	Study reference	Design/ duration	Sample size	Daily dosage range	Mean daily dose (± SD)	Outcome
Opioid antagonists						
Naltrexone (ReVia)	Kim et al. 2001a	Parallel design, 12 weeks, 1-week placebo lead-in	89 enrolled, 45 completers (20 naltrexone and 25 placebo)	50–250 mg	188 mg (±96)	Naltrexone group significantly improved compared with placebo group on CGI and G-SAS.
Mood stabilizers						
Lithium carbonate SR (Lithobid SR)	Hollander et al. 2002	Parallel design, 10 weeks	40 bipolar spectrum patients enrolled, 29 completers (12 lithium and 17 placebo)	300–900 mg	Not reported	Lithium group significantly improved compared with placebo group on CGI, PG-YBOCS, and CARS-M; 11 of 12 lithium completers responded.

Table 13–1. Double-blind, placebo-controlled trials in pathological gambling (*continued*)

Drug (trade name)	Study reference	Design/ duration	Sample size	Daily dosage range	Mean daily dose (± SD)	Outcome
Antipsychotics						
Olanzapine (Zyprexa)	Rugle 2000	Parallel design, 7 weeks	23 video poker gamblers enrolled, 21 completers (9 olanzapine and 12 placebo)	10 mg	10 mg (±0)	No significant difference was found between olanzapine and placebo groups.

Note. CARS-M=Clinician-Administered Rating Scale for Mania; CGI=Clinical Global Impressions Scale; G-SAS=Gambling Symptom Assessment Scale; PG-CGI=pathological gambling version of the Clinical Global Impressions Scale; PG-YBOCS=Yale-Brown Obsessive-Compulsive Scale modified for pathological gambling; SSRI=selective serotonin reuptake inhibitor.

placebo lead-in phase followed by an 8-week single-blind fluvoxamine trial. Seven of the 10 completers receiving fluvoxamine were found to be treatment responders, with more than 25% decreases in gambling behavior scores on the pathological gambling modification of the Yale-Brown Obsessive-Compulsive Scale (PG-YBOCS) (see Appendix E), and scores of "very much improved" or "much improved" on the Clinical Global Impressions (CGI) Scale. Of note, 2 of the 3 fluvoxamine nonresponders had histories of cyclothymia, which raised the possibility of fluvoxamine-related symptom exacerbation and gambling relapse.

The positive findings from the pilot study described above led to a subsequent double-blind crossover trial with fluvoxamine (100–250 mg/day at end point) and placebo in patients with pathological gambling (Hollander et al. 2000b). Entry criteria included a DSM-IV (American Psychiatric Association 1994) diagnosis of pathological gambling and a score of 5 or above on the South Oaks Gambling Screen (SOGS). Fifteen patients entered a 7-day placebo phase, followed by 6 patients continuing to receive placebo for 8 weeks and then fluvoxamine for the following 8 weeks. Four other patients received the medication in the reverse order. Positive response, as determined by change on the Improvement scale of the pathological gambling version of the CGI Scale (PG-CGI) after treatment, was significantly greater for fluvoxamine (40.6%) than for placebo (16.6%). As measured by changes in PG-YBOCS scores, fluvoxamine did not differ from placebo when both phases were combined. Of note, there was a phase order by treatment interaction, such that the two treatments did not statistically separate in the first phase of the crossover but did statistically separate in the second phase of the crossover trial. This finding suggests that the early placebo response rate in pathological gambling may have been transient, that the active drug effect may have been sustained, and that longer trials may be the optimal study design.

The average fluvoxamine dosage at the end point was 195 mg/day. Side effects that occurred with fluvoxamine but not with placebo included gastrointestinal distress, sedation, mild anxiety, sexual dysfunction, insomnia, light-headedness, headache, dry mouth, and increased urinary frequency. These side effects were of mild intensity, consistent with selective serotonin reuptake inhibitor (SSRI) treatment, and were not associated with early withdrawal from the study.

Another group conducted an independent double-blind, placebo-controlled study of fluvoxamine (200 mg/day) in pathological gambling in 32 patients for a longer duration of 6 months (Blanco et al. 2002). Outcome measures were reductions in money and time spent gambling per week. Overall, fluvoxamine treatment was not found to result in significant improvement over placebo treatment except in male patients and in younger patients. A high placebo response rate of 59% was found in this study. Interpretation of the findings is complicated by the high proportion of noncompleters (see Table 13–1).

These studies suggest the use of fluvoxamine dosages between 100 and 250 mg/day. Potential side effects of fluvoxamine include gastrointestinal distress, sedation, mild anxiety, sexual dysfunction, insomnia, light-headedness, and headache, which are also found with other SSRIs. Fluvoxamine acts as an inhibitor of the cytochrome P450 enzymes CYP1A2, CYP2A3/4, and CYP2C19 and therefore has the potential for some drug interactions. A controlled-release formulation of fluvoxamine has been studied in other conditions.

Paroxetine

Kim et al. (2002) performed a double-blind, placebo-controlled study with paroxetine (20–60 mg/day) in patients with pathological gambling. Patients met DSM-IV diagnostic criteria for pathological gambling, and comorbid Axis I diagnoses were excluded by the Structured Clinical Interview for DSM-III-R (SCID). Other entry requirements included a SOGS score of 5 or above. Forty-five patients completed a 1-week placebo lead-in period followed by an 8-week double-blind, placebo-controlled trial with paroxetine. The study medication was started at 20 mg/day, and the dosage was increased gradually to a maximum of 60 mg/day.

Statistically significant greater reductions in total scores on the Gambling Symptom Assessment Scale (G-SAS) (see Appendix C) were found in the paroxetine group compared with the placebo group at weeks 6 ($P=0.003$), 7 ($P=0.003$), and 8 ($P=0.042$). Statistically significant greater improvements on CGI Improvement scale scores were also found in the paroxetine group compared with the placebo group at weeks 6 ($P=0.033$), 7 ($P=0.014$), and 8 ($P=0.025$). A significantly greater proportion of patients in the paroxetine group were considered responders at weeks 7 ($P=0.011$) and 8 ($P=0.010$).

A report of a multicenter, 16-week trial of paroxetine in pathological gambling was recently published (Grant et al. 2003). No statistically significant differences were observed between the paroxetine and placebo groups on end-of-study outcome measures, including the CGI Scale, PG-YBOCS, and G-SAS scores. Notably, placebo response increased over the 16-week trial duration, and, by the end of the study, 48% of the placebo group and 59% of the paroxetine group were considered to be responders.

Similar to the double-blind studies described above, dosages of paroxetine were in the range of 20–60 mg/day. Paroxetine is usually started at 10–20 mg/day, and the dosage is increased by 20 mg/day each month if partial response occurs, up to 80 mg/day. Paroxetine may have sedative properties (which distinguish it from the other SSRIs) and is therefore often administered at nighttime. Its mild anticholinergic and antihistaminergic properties may contribute to sedation and may also lead to constipation and weight gain. At a dosage above 40 mg/day, some patients may require twice-a-day dosing. A controlled-release formulation of paroxetine is now available.

Citalopram

An open-label study was conducted with citalopram (mean dosage, 34.7 mg/day) in 15 patients with pathological gambling. Improvement was found on all gambling measures, and 13 subjects were rated as responders on the Improvement scale of the clinician-rated PG-CGI (Zimmerman et al. 2002). Of note, open-label trials do not control for placebo response, and therefore the actual effect of citalopram cannot be calculated. A stereoisomer version of the racemic citalopram, S-citalopram, is available.

Clomipramine

In a case report by our group, a 31-year-old woman with pathological gambling responded to clomipramine in a double-blind, placebo-controlled trial. The patient first received placebo for 10 weeks with minimal improvement, but with clomipramine treatment of 125 mg/day she was rated as very much improved (CGI Improvement scale score of 1), with a self-report of 90% improvement (Hollander et al. 1992).

Other Antidepressants

Nefazodone

Nefazodone, a phenylpiperazine antidepressant, acts predominantly as a 5-hydroxytryptamine type 2A (5-HT_{2A}) receptor antagonist but also has mixed serotonin/norepinephrine reuptake inhibitor properties. Nefazodone (mean dosage, 200 mg/day) has been reported to reduce the frequency of sexual obsessions and compulsions in patients with non-paraphilic sexual compulsion (Coleman et al. 2000). In an 8-week open-label study with nefazodone in 12 patients with pathological gambling, significant improvements were found on all gambling outcome measures (Pallanti et al. 2002a). Furthermore, 9 (75%) of 12 patients were rated as responders as measured by reductions in PG-YBOCS scores of 25% or greater and by PG-CGI Improvement scale scores of 1 (very much improved) or 2 (much improved). However, lack of a placebo arm in this study limits the ability to evaluate the efficacy of nefazodone in treating pathological gambling.

Opioid Antagonists

The opiate antagonist naltrexone blocks the effects of endogenous endorphins on central opiate receptors and also inhibits dopamine release in the nucleus accumbens, involving reward, pleasure, and urge mechanisms. Naltrexone has been reported to be effective in treating urge-related disorders such as alcohol dependence, obsessive-compulsive disorder, bulimia nervosa, kleptomania, and self-injurious behaviors (Crockford and el-Guebaly 1998a; Grant and Kim 2002; Keuler et al. 1996; Roth et al. 1996; Volpicelli et al. 1992). Naltrexone (100 mg/day) was found to reduce gambling and shopping urges in a 55-year-old man with a diagnosis of pathological gambling and compulsive shopping (Kim 1998). Kim and colleagues recently conducted two other studies in pathological gambling. In a 6-week open-label study with naltrexone in 17 patients with pathological gambling, naltrexone reduced urges to gamble and gambling behavior (average dosage, 157 mg/day). The majority of response occurred by the end of the fourth week (Kim and Grant 2001).

An 11-week double-blind, placebo-controlled trial with naltrexone was performed in pathological gamblers (Kim et al. 2001a). Eighty-three patients with DSM-IV diagnoses of pathological gambling and without non-nicotine-related comorbid conditions (evaluated by the SCID) were enrolled. A 1-week placebo lead-in phase was followed by 11 weeks of double-blind treatment. The dosage of the study medication was adjusted upward to 250 mg/day as needed, and the average naltrexone dosage at the end point of the study was 188 mg/day. Of the 45 completers, 75% of patients taking naltrexone showed significant improvement on both CGI patient- and clinician-rated scales compared with 24% of those completers receiving placebo (Kim et al. 2001a). Trials with other opiate antagonists are currently under way.

A common potential adverse effect of naltrexone is nausea, which may be minimized by giving the medication with food or starting at a low dosage such as 25 mg/day. Other potential side effects include insomnia, dizziness, and headache. Liver enzymes should be monitored in patients taking naltrexone, and naltrexone is contraindicated in patients with significant liver disease. Kim et al. (2001b) reported an association between elevation of liver enzymes and concurrent use of naltrexone and a nonsteroidal anti-inflammatory drug such as aspirin or ibuprofen, and consequently this combination is not recommended.

Mood Stabilizers

Mood stabilizers are effective treatments for mania. Recent studies have also demonstrated the effectiveness of both lithium carbonate (Christenson et al. 1991) and valproate (Donovan et al. 1997; Hollander et al. 2001, 2003) for the treatment of other impulsive disorders such as borderline personality disorder, disruptive behavior, and hair pulling. The impulsivity of pathological gambling clinically resembles that of bipolar disorder, and it has been suggested that impulse control disorders and bipolar spectrum disorders may be related (McElroy et al. 1996). Furthermore, comorbidity between pathological gambling and bipolar disorder has been estimated to be as high as 30% (Hollander et al. 2000a). A broader bipolar spectrum has been proposed to include bipolar I disorder, bipolar II disorder, cyclothymia, and mixed and rapid-cycling states of illness (Akiskal and Pinto 1999). Specific instruments for the diagnostic assessment of the bipolar spectrum and of subclinical and subthreshold expressions of bipolar disorder have also been developed (Benazzi and Akiskal 2003; Cassano et al. 1999; Hirschfeld et al. 2000).

Carbamazepine, an antiepileptic compound demonstrated to be effective in bipolar disorder, was studied in a placebo-controlled fashion in a single case of chronic pathological gambling and demonstrated clinical benefits at a dosage of 600 mg/day (Haller and Hinterhuber 1994). Moskowitz (1980) found lithium to be effective in three patients with pathological gambling who had comorbid bipolar features.

A recent study by our group evaluated the safety and efficacy of lithium and valproate in nonbipolar pathological gamblers (Pallanti et al. 2002b). In this 14-week single-blind trial with lithium ($n=23$) or valproate ($n=19$), patients were randomly assigned to one of the two standardized treatments. Fifteen subjects receiving lithium and 16 subjects receiving valproate treatment completed the 14-week protocol. Group 1 received 600 mg of lithium carbonate daily for days 1–4 and 900 mg/day for days 5–9. Lithium dosage was then adjusted to 1,200 mg/day according to tolerability (plasma lithium level below 1.0 mEq/L). Group 2 received 600 mg of valproate daily for days 1–5, and dosage was then adjusted to 1,500 mg/day according to tolerability and plasma drug level (50–100 mg/mL). At the end point, both lithium and valproate groups showed significant ($P<0.01$) improvement in mean scores on the PG-YBOCS, and improvement did not significantly differ between groups. Fourteen (60.9%) of the 23 patients receiving lithium and 13

(68.4%) of the 19 patients receiving valproate were responders according to scores on the CGI Improvement scale of much improved or very much improved.

Our group recently completed a 10-week double-blind, placebo-controlled trial of sustained-release lithium carbonate versus placebo in 29 bipolar spectrum pathological gamblers (Hollander et al. 2002). Bipolar spectrum disorders were defined as including DSM-IV-TR (American Psychiatric Association 2000) diagnoses of bipolar II disorder, bipolar disorder not otherwise specified, and cyclothymia, and mood swings that occurred at times unrelated to gambling urges or behavior. Bipolar spectrum patients with pathological gambling improved significantly when taking sustained-release lithium carbonate compared with placebo as measured by overall scores on the PG-YBOCS ($P=0.002$) (including scores on both Thoughts/Urges [$P=0.002$] and Behavior [$P=0.034$] subscales), PG-CGI Severity scores ($P=0.045$), and control over gambling behavior (pathological gambling self-report scale). According to scores on the PG-CGI Improvement scale, 11 (91.7%) of 12 patients receiving lithium were responders, versus 6 (35.3%) of 17 receiving placebo ($P=0.002$). Significant improvements were also found on the Total and Mania subscales of the Clinician-Administered Rating Scale for Mania, and the improvement in impulsive gambling significantly correlated with improvement in mania ratings ($r=0.478$, $P=0.009$). This suggests that reducing affective instability in such patients may help to reduce impulsive gambling.

In the double-blind, placebo-controlled trial with sustained-release lithium, the dosage range was 300–900 mg/day. Potential side effects of lithium include gastrointestinal distress, tremor, weight gain, polyuria, cognitive changes, and hypothyroidism. Renal and thyroid function should be monitored in patients taking lithium. Serum lithium levels are checked (after 5 days) during titration periods and periodically during monitoring. Therapeutic lithium levels are in the range of 0.6–1.2 mEq/L.

Atypical Antipsychotics

Given the neurobiological evidence for dopaminergic and serotonergic involvement in pathological gambling and the ability of atypical antipsychotics to target dopamine D_2 and serotonin $5\text{-}HT_2$ receptors, the potential of atypical antipsychotics in the treatment of pathological gambling has been explored. Potenza and Chambers (2001) reported the case of a 31-year-old woman with schizophrenia, nicotine dependence, and pathological gambling who had remission of her gambling and psychotic symptoms after initiation of olanzapine after inpatient hospitalization.

Improvement in symptoms also correlated temporally with the introduction of psychosocial intervention targeted at pathological gambling.

In an independent 7-week placebo-controlled trial of olanzapine in the treatment of pathological gambling without co-occurring psychotic symptoms, no differences were found between the olanzapine and placebo groups (Rugle 2000) on measures of changes in gambling urges or behavior, although differences in severity between the two groups at the beginning of the study complicates interpretation of the findings (Potenza et al. 2002). Further research is needed to investigate the efficacy and tolerability of atypical antipsychotics in the treatment of groups of pathological gamblers.

Comorbid Conditions

Patients with pathological gambling often have other co-occurring conditions (Crockford and el-Guebaly 1998b; Cunningham-Williams et al. 1998). Data from the St. Louis Epidemiologic Catchment Area Study revealed that compared with nongamblers, problem gamblers were more likely to have major depression, schizophrenia, phobias, antisocial personality disorder, alcoholism, nicotine dependence, and somatization "syndrome" (Cunningham-Williams et al. 1998). In a review of psychiatric comorbidity in pathological gambling (Crockford and el-Guebaly 1998b), patients with pathological gambling were frequently found to have comorbid substance use disorders. Less frequent comorbidities included antisocial personality disorder and major mood disorders. Bipolar disorder (Hollander et al. 2000a; McCormick et al. 1984; McElroy et al. 1996) and ADHD (Specker et al. 1995) have also been cited as being comorbid with pathological gambling.

Empirically validated data on effective treatments for individuals with pathological gambling and co-occurring disorders are limited. Therefore, the following treatment recommendations are based on these limited data and on our clinical experience. Optimal treatment for pathological gambling requires a careful diagnostic evaluation and targeting of associated or comorbid conditions that may influence gambling. These comorbid conditions may be present currently or within the patient's lifetime. Opiate antagonists such as naltrexone have been found to be effective in alcohol dependence and may provide treatment for the urges of both conditions when comorbid (Crockford and el-Guebaly 1998a). SSRIs may be effective for patients with comorbid depression and anxiety, and nefazodone may help gamblers with anxiety and depression. If bipolar spectrum symptoms are present and occur at times independent of gambling urges or behaviors, it is our recommendation to stabilize mood first, because pathological gambling symptoms may respond solely to a mood stabilizer such as lithium or valproate. For patients with comorbid ADHD and pathological gambling, bupropion, serotonin/norepineph-rine reuptake inhibitors such as high-dose venlafaxine, or stimulants may conceivably target both conditions, although no controlled data exist supporting or refuting these approaches. Figure 13–1 provides a pro-posed treatment algorithm for pathological gambling and co-occurring disorders.

Conclusion

Some promising results have emerged from pharmacological treatment studies, particularly placebo-controlled studies of serotonin reuptake in-hibitors, opiate antagonists, and mood stabilizers. Some studies, notably including a multicenter, placebo-controlled trial, have failed to replicate some earlier positive findings, possibly owing to high placebo response rates. Additional large double-blind, placebo-controlled trials are needed, and issues involving study design, outcome measures, and subject selec-tion are critical. Treatment should ultimately target all symptom domains in individual patients, including common comorbid conditions such as bi-polar spectrum disorders, ADHD, and substance abuse and dependence disorders.

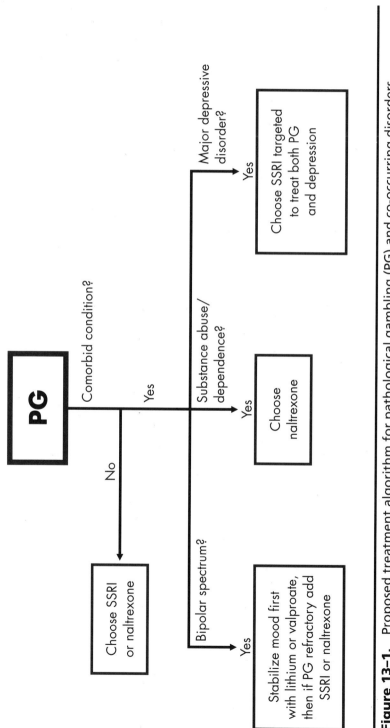

Figure 13–1. Proposed treatment algorithm for pathological gambling (PG) and co-occurring disorders.

Note. SSRI=selective serotonin reuptake inhibitor.

References

Akiskal HS, Pinto O: The evolving bipolar spectrum. Prototypes I, II, III, and IV. Psychiatr Clin North Am 22:517–534, 1999

American Psychiatric Association: Diagnostic and Statistical Manual of Mental Disorders, 4th Edition. Washington, DC, American Psychiatric Association, 1994

American Psychiatric Association: Diagnostic and Statistical Manual of Mental Disorders, 4th Edition, Text Revision. Washington, DC, American Psychiatric Association, 2000

Benazzi F, Akiskal HS: Refining the evaluation of bipolar II: beyond the strict SCID-CV guidelines for hypomania. J Affect Disord 73:33–38, 2003

Bergh C, Eklund T, Sodersten P, et al: Altered dopamine function in pathological gambling. Psychol Med 27:473–475, 1997

Blanco C, Orensanz-Munoz L, Blanco-Jerez C, et al: Pathological gambling and platelet MAO activity: a psychobiological study. Am J Psychiatry 153:119–121, 1996

Blanco C, Petkova E, Ibáñez A, et al: A pilot placebo-controlled study of fluvoxamine for pathological gambling. Ann Clin Psychiatry 14:9–15, 2002

Cassano GB, Dell'Osso L, Frank E, et al: The bipolar spectrum: a clinical reality in search of diagnostic criteria and an assessment methodology. J Affect Disord 54:319–328, 1999

Christenson GA, Popkin MK, Mackenzie TB, et al: Lithium treatment of chronic hair pulling. J Clin Psychiatry 52:116–120, 1991

Coleman E, Gratzer T, Nesvacil L, et al: Nefazodone and the treatment of nonparaphilic compulsive sexual behavior: a retrospective study. J Clin Psychiatry 61:282–284, 2000

Comings DE: The molecular genetics of pathological gambling. CNS Spectr 3:20–37, 1998

Crockford DN, el-Guebaly N: Naltrexone in the treatment of pathological gambling and alcohol dependence (letter). Can J Psychiatry 43:86, 1998a

Crockford DN, el-Guebaly N: Psychiatric comorbidity in pathological gambling: a critical review. Can J Psychiatry 43:43–50, 1998b

Cunningham-Williams RM, Cottler LB, Compton WM III, et al: Taking chances: problem gamblers and mental health disorders—results from the St. Louis Epidemiologic Catchment Area Study. Am J Public Health 88:1093–1096, 1998

DeCaria CM, Hollander E, Grossman R, et al: Diagnosis, neurobiology, and treatment of pathological gambling. J Clin Psychiatry 57 (suppl 8):80–83, 1996

DeCaria CM, Begaz T, Hollander E: Serotonergic and noradrenergic function in pathological gambling. CNS Spectr 3:38–47, 1998

Donovan SJ, Susser ES, Nunes EV, et al: Divalproex treatment of disruptive adolescents: a report of 10 cases. J Clin Psychiatry 58:12–15, 1997

Grant JE, Kim SW: An open-label study of naltrexone in the treatment of kleptomania. J Clin Psychiatry 63:349–356, 2002

Grant JE, Kim SW, Potenza MN, et al: Paroxetine treatment of pathological gambling: a multi-centre randomized controlled trial. Int Clin Psychopharmacol 18:243–249, 2003

Haller R, Hinterhuber H: Treatment of pathological gambling with carbamazepine (letter). Pharmacopsychiatry 27:129, 1994

Hirschfeld RM, Williams JB, Spitzer RL, et al: Development and validation of a screening instrument for bipolar spectrum disorder: the Mood Disorder Questionnaire. Am J Psychiatry 157:1873–1875, 2000

Hollander E: Introduction, in Obsessive-Compulsive–Related Disorders. Edited by Hollander E. Washington, DC, American Psychiatric Press, 1993, p 2

Hollander E: Treatment of obsessive-compulsive spectrum disorders with SSRIs. Br J Psychiatry 173:7–12, 1998

Hollander E, Pallanti S: Current and experimental therapeutics of obsessive-compulsive disorder, in Neuropsychopharmacology: The Fifth Generation of Progress: An Official Publication of the American College of Neuropsychopharmacology. Edited by Davis KL, Charney D, Coyle JT, et al. Philadelphia, PA, Lippincott Williams & Wilkins, 2002, pp 1647–1664

Hollander E, Frenkel M, DeCaria C, et al: Treatment of pathological gambling with clomipramine (letter). Am J Psychiatry 149:710–711, 1992

Hollander E, DeCaria CM, Mari E, et al: Short-term single-blind fluvoxamine treatment of pathological gambling. Am J Psychiatry 155:1781–1783, 1998

Hollander E, Allen A, Kwon J: Clomipramine vs desipramine crossover trial in body dysmorphic disorder: selective efficacy of a serotonin reuptake inhibitor in imagined ugliness. Arch Gen Psychiatry 56:1033–1039, 1999

Hollander E, Buchalter AJ, DeCaria CM: Pathological gambling. Psychiatr Clin North Am 23:629–642, 2000a

Hollander E, DeCaria CM, Finkell JN, et al: A randomized double-blind fluvoxamine/placebo crossover trial in pathologic gambling. Biol Psychiatry 47:813–817, 2000b

Hollander E, Allen A, Lopez RP, et al: A preliminary double-blind placebo controlled trial of divalproex sodium in borderline personality disorder. J Clin Psychiatry 62:199–203, 2001

Hollander E, Pallanti S, Baldini-Rossi N, et al: Sustained release lithium/placebo treatment response in bipolar spectrum pathological gamblers. Poster presented at the 42nd Annual New Clinical Drug Evaluation Unit Meeting, Boca Raton, FL, June 10–13, 2002

Hollander E, Tracy KA, Swann A, et al: Divalproex in the treatment of impulsive aggression: efficacy in cluster B personality disorders. Neuropsychopharmacology 28:1186–1197, 2003

Johannessen CU: Mechanisms of action of valproate: a commentatory. Neurochem Int 37:103–110, 2000

Keuler DJ, Altemus M, Michelson D, et al: Behavioral effects of naloxone infusion in obsessive-compulsive disorder. Biol Psychiatry 40:154–156, 1996

Kim SW: Opioid antagonists in the treatment of impulse-control disorders. J Clin Psychiatry 59:159–164, 1998

Kim SW, Grant JE: An open naltrexone treatment study in pathological gambling disorder. Int Clin Psychopharmacol 16:285–289, 2001

Kim SW, Grant JE, Adson DE, et al: Double-blind naltrexone and placebo comparison study in the treatment of pathological gambling. Biol Psychiatry 49:914–921, 2001a

Kim SW, Grant JE, Adson DE, et al: A preliminary report on possible naltrexone and nonsteroidal analgesic interactions (letter). J Clin Psychopharmacol 21:632–634, 2001b

Kim SW, Grant JE, Adson DE, et al: A double-blind placebo-controlled study of the efficacy and safety of paroxetine in the treatment of pathological gambling. J Clin Psychiatry 63:501–507, 2002

McCormick RA, Russo AM, Ramirez LF, et al: Affective disorders among pathological gamblers seeking treatment. Am J Psychiatry 141:215–218, 1984

McElroy SL, Pope HG Jr, Keck PE Jr, et al: Are impulse-control disorders related to bipolar disorder? Compr Psychiatry 37:229–240, 1996

Moreno I, Saiz-Ruiz J, Lopez-Ibor JJ: Serotonin and gambling dependence. Hum Psychopharmacol 6 (suppl):S9–S12, 1991

Moskowitz JA: Lithium and lady luck: use of lithium carbonate in compulsive gambling. N Y State J Med 80:785–788, 1980

Pallanti S, Baldini Rossi N, Sood E, et al: Nefazodone treatment of pathological gambling: a prospective open-label controlled trial. J Clin Psychiatry 63:1034–1039, 2002a

Pallanti S, Quercioli L, Sood E, et al: Lithium and valproate treatment of pathological gambling: a randomized single-blind study. J Clin Psychiatry 63:559–564, 2002b

Perez de Castro I, Ibáñez A, Torres P, et al: Genetic association study between pathological gambling and a functional DNA polymorphism at the D4 receptor gene. Pharmacogenetics 7:345–348, 1997

Phillips KA, Albertini RS, Rasmussen SA: A randomized placebo-controlled trial of fluoxetine in body dysmorphic disorder. Arch Gen Psychiatry 59:381–388, 2002

Potenza MN, Chambers RA: Schizophrenia and pathological gambling. Am J Psychiatry 158:497–498, 2001

Potenza MN, Fiellin DA, Heninger GR, et al: Gambling: an addictive behavior with health and primary care implications. J Gen Intern Med 17:721–731, 2002

Roth AS, Ostroff RB, Hoffman RE: Naltrexone as a treatment for repetitive self-injurious behavior: an open-label trial. J Clin Psychiatry 57:233–237, 1996

Roy A, Custer R, Lorenz V, et al: Depressed pathological gamblers. Acta Psychiatr Scand 77:163–165, 1988

Rugle L: The use of olanzapine in the treatment of video poker pathological gamblers. Poster presented at the 1st annual conference of the National Center for Responsible Gaming, Las Vegas, NV, December 3–5, 2000

Specker SM, Carlson GA, Christenson GA, et al: Impulse control disorders and attention deficit disorder in pathological gamblers. Ann Clin Psychiatry 7:175–179, 1995

Volpicelli JR, Alterman AI, Hayashida M, et al: Naltrexone in the treatment of alcohol dependence. Arch Gen Psychiatry 49:876–880, 1992

Zimmerman M, Breen RB, Posternak MA: An open-label study of citalopram in the treatment of pathological gambling. J Clin Psychiatry 63:44–48, 2002

Chapter 14

Screening and Assessment Instruments

Randy Stinchfield, Ph.D., L.P.
Richard Govoni, Ph.D.
G. Ron Frisch, Ph.D., C.Psych.

In this chapter, we describe instruments currently available for assessment of adults with pathological gambling and provide information on the development, content, intended purpose, psychometric properties (reliability, validity, and classification accuracy), norms, administration methods, scoring, and interpretation of each instrument. See also the Appendix at the end of this chapter for a synopsis of instruments.

Screening and Diagnostic Instruments

South Oaks Gambling Screen

The South Oaks Gambling Screen (SOGS; Lesieur and Blume 1987) is a 20-item self-report screening instrument for pathological gambling (see Appendix D). DSM-III (American Psychiatric Association 1980) and DSM-III-R (American Psychiatric Association 1987) diagnostic criteria were used in the development and validation of the SOGS (Culleton 1989; Lesieur and Blume 1987). The SOGS is scored by summing selected items, with a score of 5 or more indicating probable pathological gambling. The SOGS has demonstrated excellent internal consistency (Cronbach $\alpha=0.97$) and 1-month test-retest reliability ($r=0.71$). Validity was examined by correlating the SOGS with counselors' independent assessments ($r=0.86$), family member assessment ($r=0.60$), and DSM-III-R pathological gambling diagnosis ($r=0.94$). The SOGS was compared with DSM-III-R diagnosis of pathological gambling and demonstrated satisfactory overall diagnostic accuracy among Gamblers Anonymous members (98.1%), university students (95.3%), and hospital employees (99.3%). The original SOGS is based on lifetime gambling activity and does not differentiate pathological gamblers in remission from those actively gambling problematically.

Little systematic research has been conducted on the psychometric properties of the SOGS under varying conditions of use, such as estimating the prevalence of pathological gambling in the general population. Also, psychometric data obtained in the development of the SOGS are now almost 20 years old and diagnostic criteria for pathological gambling have undergone revision, raising questions regarding the psychometric properties of the SOGS within a current context.

The SOGS recently demonstrated satisfactory reliability and validity for a 1-year time frame (Stinchfield 2002). Satisfactory reliability was demonstrated in general (Cronbach $\alpha=0.69$) and treatment samples (Cronbach $\alpha=0.86$). Satisfactory validity was observed between the SOGS and DSM-IV criteria (American Psychiatric Association 1994) ($r=0.77$ in the general sample and $r=0.83$ in the treatment sample). Correlations with other gambling problem severity measures in the gambling treatment sample were moderate to high (ranging from $r=0.33$ to $r=0.65$). The SOGS demonstrated high overall diagnostic accuracy (0.96), high sensitivity (0.99), modest specificity (0.75), high positive predictive power (0.96), high negative predictive power (0.90), and low false-positive (0.04) and low-false negative rates (0.10). The SOGS showed poorer classification accuracy in the general population, with a modest sensitivity rate of 0.67 and a high false-positive rate of 0.50 (Stinchfield 2002), further raising questions regarding its widespread use in prevalence estimate studies. The SOGS overestimated the number of pathological gamblers in the general population compared with DSM-IV criteria.

Ladouceur and colleagues (2000) examined the accuracy of the SOGS in terms of how well children, adolescents, and adults understand the items and the effect that misunderstanding item content has on scores. Most participants misunderstood some SOGS items, leading to higher scores. Clarification of misunderstood items resulted in lower SOGS scores and fewer respondents being classified as probable pathological gamblers.

Gamblers Anonymous 20 Questions

Gamblers Anonymous (GA) disseminates 20 questions (GA-20) for the purpose of identifying problem gamblers (view the questions on its Web site, http://www.gamblersanonymous.org/20questions.html). A score of 7 or more affirmative answers indicates that the respondent is a problem gambler. Although the GA-20 correlates with gambling frequency (Kuley and Jacobs 1988), only two studies have reported psychometric information. In one, the GA-20 demonstrated high internal consistency (Cronbach $\alpha=0.94$) and correlation with the SOGS ($r=0.94$) (Ursua and Uribelarrea 1998). The GA-20 differentiated between problem gamblers and social gamblers with a sensitivity of 0.98, specificity of 0.99, and overall diagnostic accuracy of 0.99. These findings are based on a sample with a base rate of approximately 50%, inflating classification accuracy indices.

Massachusetts Gambling Screen

The Massachusetts Gambling Screen (MAGS) was designed to screen for gambling problems and assess problem gambling among adolescents and adults (Shaffer et al. 1994). The MAGS measures past-year behavior and includes 14 items adapted from the Short Michigan Alcoholism Screening Test (Selzer et al. 1975). The MAGS classifies respondents as nonproblem, in-transition, or pathological gamblers using a weighted scoring derived from a discriminant function analysis. In terms of validity, the MAGS total discriminant score correlated ($r=0.83$) with the total DSM-IV score.

DSM-IV Multiple Response

Fisher (2000b) developed a 10-item questionnaire, the DSM-IV Multiple Response (DSM-IV-MR), to measure DSM-IV diagnostic criteria of pathological gambling in adults. There is 1 item for each criterion, and items are paraphrased from DSM-IV criteria. Most items have four response options: 1) never, 2) once or twice, 3) sometimes, and 4) often. Each item is allocated 1 point, and scores range from 0 to 10. A person with a score of 3 or 4—including at least 1 point from criterion 8, 9, or 10—is classified as a problem gambler, and a person with a score of 5 or more is classified as a severe problem gambler. The DSM-IV-MR has satisfactory internal consistency reliability (Cronbach $\alpha=0.79$). In terms of validity, significantly different mean scores were found between regular and nonregular gamblers and between self-identified problem gamblers and social gamblers.

Diagnostic Interview for Gambling Schedule

The Diagnostic Interview for Gambling Schedule (DIGS) is a structured clinical interview (Winters et al. 2002). In addition to 20 diagnostic symptom items (lifetime and past year), the DIGS evaluates gambling treatment history, onset of gambling, and family and social functioning. The DSM-IV diagnostic criteria items demonstrated good internal consistency (Cronbach $\alpha=0.92$). The total diagnostic score (range, 0–10) exhibited moderate correlations with the following measures of gambling severity: gambling frequency ($r=0.39$), highest amount gambled in 1 day ($r=0.42$), current gambling debt ($r=0.47$), number of financial problems ($r=0.40$), number of borrowing sources ($r=0.31$), and legal problems ($r=0.50$).

National Opinion Research Center DSM-IV Screen for Gambling Problems

A U.S. national gambling survey was conducted in 1998 by the National Opinion Research Center (1999) using the National Opinion Research Center DSM-IV Screen for Gambling Problems (NODS). The NODS includes 17 questions reflecting DSM-IV diagnostic criteria. Interpretation of NODS scores for respondents who have gambled and lost more than $100 is as follows: a score of 0 designates a low-risk gambler, a score of 1 or 2 indicates an at-risk gambler, a score of 3 or 4 designates a problem gambler, and a score of 5 or greater indicates a pathological gambler.

    In a clinical sample of 40 individuals in outpatient problem gambling treatment, the NODS demonstrated high test-retest coefficients for lifetime ($r=0.99$) and past-year gambling ($r=0.98$).

Lie/Bet Questionnaire

The Lie/Bet Questionnaire is a two-item screen for pathological gambling (Johnson et al. 1997): 1) "Have you ever had to lie to people important to you about how much you gambled?" and 2) "Have you ever felt the need to bet more and more money?" This two-item screen has demonstrated a sensitivity of 0.99, specificity of 0.91, positive predictive power of 0.92, and negative predictive power of 0.99 in comparing Gamblers Anonymous members and control subjects who were not problem gamblers. In a second study, the questionnaire demonstrated a sensitivity of 1.00, specificity of 0.85, positive predictive power of 0.78, and negative predictive power of 1.00 (Johnson et al. 1998).

Gambling Assessment Module

The Gambling Assessment Module (GAM-IV) is in early stages of test-ing, and little psychometric information is available (Cunningham-Williams et al. 2003). Multiple versions of the GAM-IV exist for dif-ferent administration methodologies, including interview with paper and pencil, interview with computer, and self-administration. The GAM-IV generates DSM-IV diagnoses for seven different types of gam-bling. Good agreement exists between the GAM-IV and clinician rat-ings for five diagnostic criteria ($\kappa=0.5-0.7$), but the remaining five criteria had poor agreement ($\kappa=0.0-0.3$) (Cunningham-Williams et al. 2003).

Gambling Behavior Interview

The Gambling Behavior Interview (GBI) is a 76-item instrument assess-ing past-year pathological gambling (Stinchfield 2002, 2003; Stinchfield et al., submitted). The GBI consists of eight content domains: 1) gam-bling attitudes (4 items); 2) frequency of different types of gambling (15 items); 3) time and money spent gambling (4 items); 4) gambling fre-quency at different venues (7 items); 5) the SOGS (25 items); 6) DSM-IV diagnostic criteria (10 items); 7) research diagnostic items (32 items); and 8) demographics (9 items).

The GBI has excellent internal consistency (Cronbach $\alpha=0.92$), and all 10 diagnostic criteria had high corrected item-total correlations (ranging from $r=0.52$ to $r=0.82$). DSM-IV criteria also exhibited con-struct validity with good discrimination between the general-popula-tion and gambling-treatment samples. Convergent validity of DSM-IV criteria was exhibited by generally high correlations with concurrent problem gambling severity measures (ranging from $r=0.27$ to $r=0.90$). Discriminant validity was exhibited by low correlations with variables unrelated to problem gambling (ranging from $r=-0.02$ to $r=-0.16$).

Although the standard DSM-IV cutoff score of 5 yielded respectable overall diagnostic accuracy (0.91), sensitivity was low (0.83) and the false-negative rate was high (0.13). A cutoff score of 4 yielded better clas-sification accuracy—including higher overall diagnostic accuracy (0.95), sensitivity (0.93), and specificity (0.96) and a lower false-negative rate (0.06). The discriminant function analysis yielded better classification ac-curacy than either cutoff score, with an overall diagnostic accuracy of 0.97, sensitivity of 0.94, and specificity of 0.99.

Early Intervention Gambling Health Test

The Early Intervention Gambling Health Test (EIGHT) is an eight-item screening instrument (see Appendix B) designed for use by general practitioners (Sullivan 1999; Sullivan et al., in press). If four or more questions are answered affirmatively, the person may meet criteria for pathological gambling. EIGHT scores correlated with SOGS scores ($r=0.75$) and were in good to excellent agreement with counselor-based ratings and diagnoses of pathological gambling (S. Sullivan, personal communication, May 6, 2003). When administered to 100 prison inmates, the EIGHT correlated with the SOGS ($r=0.83$), had high sensitivity (0.91) with DSM-IV diagnostic criteria, and had low specificity (0.50) and low positive predictive value (0.59) (Sullivan et al., in press).

Time-Line Follow-Back

The Time-Line Follow-Back (TLFB) (Sobell et al. 1985) has been adapted for assessing gambling (Hodgins and Makarchuk 2003; Stinchfield et al. 2001; Weinstock et al. 2004). The TLFB assesses the number of days and the amount of money spent gambling over a 6-month period. The TLFB has adequate 3-week test-retest reliability, with intraclass correlations of 0.61–0.98. Agreement with collaterals was fair to good, with intraclass correlations of 0.46–0.65.

   Stinchfield et al. (2001) adapted the TLFB to assess gambling over a 4-week period. The TLFB correlated with other measures of gambling frequency ($r=0.24$ to $r=0.53$) (Stinchfield et al. 2001). Weinstock and colleagues (2004) similarly generated a TLFB (G-TLFB) to evaluate young adult frequent gamblers. The G-TLFB demonstrated adequate to excellent 2-week test-retest reliability ($r=0.73$ to $r=0.93$), and scores correlated with daily self-monitoring reports ($r=0.59$ to $r=0.87$). Dimensions of frequency and duration demonstrated concurrent validity with other gambling assessments, and the G-TLFB demonstrated discriminant validity with demographic variables and a measure of positive impression management.

Addiction Severity Index for Pathological Gamblers and the Gambling Severity Index

The Addiction Severity Index (ASI) was modified for pathological gambling (ASI-PG) by Lesieur and Blume (1992) to include six gambling items that are scored to create a composite score, the Gambling Severity Index (GSI). The GSI exhibited satisfactory reliability (Cronbach

$\alpha=0.73$) and validity ($r=0.57$ with the SOGS). The GSI seems to be particularly well suited for problem gamblers with substance use problems.

Structured Clinical Interview for Pathological Gambling

The Structured Clinical Interview for Pathological Gambling (SCI-PG) is a clinician-administered, DSM-IV–based diagnostic interview that is compatible with the Structured Clinical Interview for DSM-IV (Grant et al., in press). The SCI-PG assesses both the 10 inclusion criteria and the exclusionary criterion ("not better accounted for by a manic episode") of pathological gambling. The SCI-PG demonstrated excellent reliability, validity, and classification accuracy in preliminary testing of individuals with gambling problems. Further testing is needed to examine its suitability for other populations.

Instruments for Evaluation of Treatment Efficacy

Gambling Treatment Outcome Monitoring System

The Gambling Treatment Outcome Monitoring System (GAMTOMS) is a multidimensional assessment system that includes the following instruments: 1) Gambling Treatment Admission Questionnaire, 2) Primary Discharge Questionnaire, 3) Client Follow-up Questionnaire, 4) Staff Discharge Form, 5) Significant Other Intake Questionnaire, and 6) Significant Other Follow-up Questionnaire (Stinchfield 1999; Stinchfield and Winters 1996, 2001). Reliability and validity of the GAMTOMS have been evaluated in a treatment sample of more than 1,000 patients from a Minnesota gambling treatment outcome study (Stinchfield 1999; Stinchfield and Winters 1996, 2001). The GAMTOMS has also been evaluated for reliability, validity, classification accuracy, and validity of self-reporting with a sample of 74 gambling treatment patients (Stinchfield et al. 2001). The GAMTOMS gambling frequency section demonstrated modest correlations with the gambling TLFB ($r=0.53$), the SOGS ($r=0.47$), and DSM-IV criteria ($r=0.36$).

Pathological Gambling Modification of the Yale-Brown Obsessive-Compulsive Scale

The Yale-Brown Obsessive-Compulsive Scale was modified to measure severity of pathological gambling and change in symptoms in response to treatment (PG-YBOCS) (Hollander et al. 1998) (see Appendix E). Interrater agreement on Urge and Behavior scores was high, with intraclass correlations of 0.99 and 0.98, respectively. In terms of validity, the PG-YBOCS correlated with the Clinical Global Impressions (CGI) pathological gambling scale ($r=0.89$) and the SOGS ($r=0.86$).

Gambling Symptom Assessment Scale

The Gambling Symptom Assessment Scale (G-SAS) was developed to assess gambling symptoms during treatment (Kim et al. 2001) (see Appendix C). The G-SAS measures past-week gambling urges and thoughts and includes 12 items with response options ranging from 0 to 4. Responses are summed, and the total score range is 0–48, with scores of 31 or above signifying severe symptoms; scores of 21–30 signifying moderate symptoms; and scores of 20 or less, mild symptoms. In 58 patients, the G-SAS demonstrated satisfactory 1-week test-retest reliability ($r=0.70$) and internal consistency (Cronbach $\alpha=0.89$). In terms of validity, G-SAS scores correlated with those of the CGI Improvement ($r=0.78$) and Severity ($r=0.81$) scales.

Clinical Global Impressions Scale—Pathological Gambling

The Clinical Global Impressions (CGI) Scale was developed for treatment studies of schizophrenia (Guy 1976). It contains three items that the clinician rates: severity of illness, global improvement, and treatment efficacy. The CGI Scale has been adapted by gambling researchers (Hollander et al. 1998; Kim et al. 2001) to assess severity of pathological gambling and to measure "global gambling improvement" in psychopharmacological studies. The CGI Severity and Improvement items have 7-point response options. No psychometric information on the adaptation of this scale to pathological gambling is available.

Youth Gambling Assessment Instruments

Winters and colleagues (1993, 1995) revised the SOGS for adolescents (SOGS–Revised for Adolescents [SOGS-RA]) by using a past-year time frame, changing the wording of items and response options to better reflect adolescent gambling and reading levels, eliminating two items considered to have poor content validity for adolescents, and giving only 1 point for any source of borrowed money rather than the 9 possible points for separate sources as in the SOGS. A score of 4 or more indicates a problem gambler; a score of 2–3, an at-risk gambler; and a score of 0–1, a nonproblem gambler (Winters et al. 1995).

Fisher (2000a) developed a nine-item questionnaire to measure DSM-IV diagnostic criteria of pathological gambling in juveniles. There is one item for each DSM-IV criterion, and the items are adapted from the DSM-IV criteria to reflect the developmental stage of youth. Fisher simplified the language, omitted details that were less relevant for youths, and excluded criterion 10 ("relies on others to provide money to relieve a desperate financial situation caused by gambling"). Eight of the nine scored items have four response options: 1) never, 2) once or twice, 3) sometimes, and 4) often. Scores range from 0 to 9, and a score of 4 or more identifies a problem gambler.

Conclusion

Multiple instruments have been developed in response to a need to detect and measure problem gambling. Existing instruments require additional psychometric evaluation—particularly with regard to specific population groups (such as seniors), for which new or modified instruments might be optimal. Information generated from these studies will enable clinicians and researchers to make more informed decisions as to how—within specific settings and for specific purposes—to best identify, assess, and monitor individuals with gambling problems.

References

American Psychiatric Association: Diagnostic and Statistical Manual of Mental Disorders, 3rd Edition. Washington, DC, American Psychiatric Association, 1980

American Psychiatric Association: Diagnostic and Statistical Manual of Mental Disorders, 3rd Edition, Revised. Washington, DC, American Psychiatric Association, 1987

American Psychiatric Association: Diagnostic and Statistical Manual of Mental Disorders, 4th Edition. Washington, DC, American Psychiatric Association, 1994

Culleton RP: The prevalence rates of pathological gambling: a look at methods. Journal of Gambling Behavior 5:22–41, 1989

Cunningham-Williams R, Books SJ, Cottler LB, et al: Diagnostic concordance between the GAM-IV-12 and clinician ratings among pathological gamblers in St. Louis. Paper presented at the 3rd annual conference of the National Center for Responsible Gaming, Las Vegas, NV, December 2–5, 2003

Fisher S: Developing the DSM-IV-DSM-IV criteria to identify adolescent problem gambling in non-clinical populations. J Gambl Stud 16:253–273, 2000a

Fisher S: Measuring the prevalence of sector-specific problem gambling: a study of casino patrons. J Gambl Stud 16:25–51, 2000b

Grant JE, Steinberg M, Kim SW, et al: Preliminary validity and reliability testing of a Structured Clinical Interview for Pathological Gambling (SCI-PG). Psychiatr Res (in press)

Guy W: Clinical Global Impressions, in ECDEU Assessment Manual for Psychopharmacology, Revised (DHEW Publ No ADM 76-338). Edited by Guy W. Rockville, MD, National Institute of Mental Health, Psychopharmacology Research Branch, 1976, pp 218–222

Hodgins DC, Makarchuk K: Trusting problem gamblers: reliability and validity of self-reported gambling behavior. Psychol Addict Behav 17:244–248, 2003

Hollander E, DeCaria CM, Mari E, et al: Short-term single-blind fluvoxamine treatment of pathological gambling. Am J Psychiatry 155:1781–1783, 1998

Johnson EE, Hamer R, Nora RM, et al: The Lie/Bet Questionnaire for screening pathological gamblers. Psychol Rep 80:83–88, 1997

Johnson EE, Hamer RM, Nora RM, et al: The Lie/Bet Questionnaire for screening pathological gamblers: a follow-up study. Psychol Rep 83:1219–1224, 1998

Kim SW, Grant JE, Adson DE, et al: Double-blind naltrexone and placebo comparison study in the treatment of pathological gambling. Biol Psychiatry 49:914–921, 2001

Kuley NB, Jacobs DF: The relationship between dissociative-like experiences and sensation seeking among social and problem gamblers. Journal of Gambling Behavior 4:197–207, 1988

Ladouceur R, Bouchard C, Rheaume N, et al: Is the SOGS an accurate measure of pathological gambling among children, adolescents and adults? J Gambl Stud 16:1–24, 2000

Lesieur HR, Blume SB: The South Oaks Gambling Screen (SOGS): a new instrument for the identification of pathological gamblers. Am J Psychiatry 144:1184–1188, 1987

Lesieur HR, Blume SB: Modifying the Addiction Severity Index for use with pathological gamblers. Am J Addict 1:240–247, 1992

National Opinion Research Center: Gambling Impact and Behavior Study: Report to the National Gambling Impact Study Commission. Chicago, IL, National Opinion Research Center at the University of Chicago, 1999. Available at: http://www.norc.uchicago.edu/new/gamb-fin.htm. Accessed December 13, 2003.

Selzer ML, Vinokur A, van Rooijen L: A self-administered Short Michigan Alcoholism Screening Test (SMAST). J Stud Alcohol 36:117–126, 1975

Shaffer HJ, LaBrie R, Scanlan KM, et al: Pathological gambling among adolescents: Massachusetts Gambling Screen (MAGS). J Gambl Stud 10:339–362, 1994

Sobell LC, Sobell MB, Maisto SA, et al: Time-Line Follow-Back assessment method, in Alcoholism Treatment Assessment Research Instruments (NIAAA Treatment Handbook Series, Vol 2) (DHHS Publ No 85-1380). Edited by Lettieri DJ, Nelson JE, Sayers MA. Rockville, MD, National Institute on Alcoholism and Alcohol Abuse, 1985, pp 530–534

Stinchfield R: Gambling treatment outcome monitoring system, in Behavioral Outcomes and Guidelines Sourcebook. Edited by Coughlin KM. New York, Faulkner & Gray, 1999, pp 173–174, 464–466

Stinchfield R: Reliability, validity, and classification accuracy of the South Oaks Gambling Screen (SOGS). Addict Behav 27:1–19, 2002

Stinchfield R: Reliability, validity, and classification accuracy of a measure of DSM-IV diagnostic criteria for pathological gambling. Am J Psychiatry 160:180–182, 2003

Stinchfield R, Winters K: Effectiveness of Six State-Supported Compulsive Gambling Treatment Programs in Minnesota. Minneapolis, Compulsive Gambling Program, Mental Health Division, Minnesota Department of Human Services, 1996

Stinchfield R, Winters KC: Outcome of Minnesota's gambling treatment programs. J Gambl Stud 17:217–245, 2001

Stinchfield R, Winters KC, Botzet A, et al: Gambling Treatment Outcome Monitoring Systems (GAMTOMS): User Manual. St. Paul, MN, Minnesota Department of Human Services, 2001

Stinchfield R, Govoni R, Frisch GR: DSM-IV diagnostic criteria for pathological gambling: reliability, validity, and classification accuracy. Am J Addict (in press)

Sullivan S: Development of the "EIGHT" Problem Gambling Screen. Unpublished doctoral thesis, Auckland Medical School, Auckland, New Zealand, 1999

Sullivan S, Brown R, Skinner B: Development of a problem gambling screen for use in a prison inmate population. eGambling (in press)

Ursua MP, Uribelarrea LL: 20 questions of Gamblers Anonymous: a psychometric study with population of Spain. J Gambl Stud 14:3–15, 1998

Weinstock J, Whelan JP, Meyers AW: Behavioral assessment of gambling: an application of the timeline followback method. Psychol Assess 16:72–80, 2004

Winters KC, Stinchfield R, Fulkerson J: Toward the development of an adolescent gambling problem severity scale. J Gambl Stud 9:63–84, 1993

Winters KC, Stinchfield R, Kim L: Monitoring adolescent gambling in Minnesota. J Gambl Stud 11:165–183, 1995

Winters KC, Specker S, Stinchfield R: Measuring pathological gambling with the Diagnostic Interview for Gambling Severity (DIGS), in The Downside: Problem and Pathological Gambling. Edited by Marotta JJ, Cornelius JA, Eadington WR. Reno, NV, University of Nevada, 2002, pp 143–148

Appendix: Instruments for the Assessment of Pathological Gambling

Instrument	Content areas	Number of items	Administration time and method
Adult Instruments for Screening and Diagnosis			
South Oaks Gambling Screen (SOGS) (Lesieur and Blume 1987)	Games played; signs and symptoms of problem gambling; negative consequences; sources of money to gamble	20 scored items	10- to 20-min PPQ
Gamblers Anonymous 20 questions (GA-20) (Ursua and Uribelarrea 1998)	Signs and symptoms of compulsive gambling; negative consequences	20	10-min PPQ or interview

| | **Psychometrics** | | |
Scoring	**Reliability[†]**	**Validity**	**Classification accuracy indices**
1 point for each item Score range: 0–20 Score of 5+ indicates probable PG	$\alpha = 0.97$; 1-month TRT reliability: $r=0.71$	Correlations with counselor assessments ($r=0.86$), family member assessment ($r=0.60$), and DSM-III-R PG diagnosis ($r=0.94$)	Gamblers Anonymous (GA) members ($n=213$), university students ($n=384$), and hospital employees ($n=152$); criterion was DSM-III-R diagnosis of PG ODA among GA members=0.98, university students=0.95, and hospital employees=0.99
1 point for each item Score of 7+ indicates compulsive gambler	$\alpha = 0.94$	GA-20 yielded high correlations with frequency of gambling and with dissociative experiences; GA-20 was highly correlated with SOGS ($r=0.94$)	Criterion is group membership 127 problem gamblers 142 nonproblem social gamblers BR=0.47 Sens=0.98 Spec=0.99 ODA=0.99 Classification accuracy indices are based on sample with BR of about 50%, which inflates classification accuracy indices

Instrument	Content areas	Number of items	Administration time and method
Adult Instruments for Screening and Diagnosis *(continued)*			
Massachusetts Gambling Screen (MAGS) (Shaffer et al. 1994)	Signs and symptoms of PG; psychological and social problems associated with gambling; study also included 12-item measure of DSM-IV diagnostic criteria	14 items (7 items scored)	5- to 10-min PPQ
DSM-IV Multiple Response (DSM-IV-MR) (Fisher 2000b)	DSM-IV diagnostic criteria	10, one item for each criterion; 4-point response options for most items	5-min questionnaire
Diagnostic Interview for Gambling Schedule (DIGS) (Winters et al. 2002)	Demographics, gambling involvement, treatment history, onset of gambling, gambling frequency, amounts of money bet and lost, sources of borrowed money, financial problems, legal problems, mental health screen, other impulse control disorders, medical status, family and social functioning, and diagnostic symptoms (lifetime and past year)	20 diagnostic symptom items measure the 10 DSM-IV diagnostic criteria 2 items for each criterion	30-min interview

| | **Psychometrics** | | |
Scoring	**Reliability[†]**	**Validity**	**Classification accuracy indices**
Each of 7 MAGS items are multiplied by discriminant function coefficient, then summed and a constant is added 0–2 = transitional or potential pathological gambler 2+ = PG	MAGS 7-item scale, $\alpha = 0.84$; DSM-IV 12-item scale, $\alpha = 0.89$	MAGS total discriminant score was correlated with total DSM-IV score, $r = 0.83$	NA
1 point for each item Score range: 0–10 Score of 3–4 (including at least 1 point from criterion 8, 9, or 10) designates a problem gambler Score of 5+ indicates a severe problem gambler	$\alpha = 0.79$	Discriminated between regular and nonregular gamblers and between problem and social gamblers	NA
If respondent endorses either of two items per criterion, the criterion is considered endorsed; 1 point for each of 10 criteria Score range: 0–10 Score of 5+ indicates PG	$\alpha = 0.92$	Total diagnostic score (0–10) exhibited significant correlations with the following measures of gambling problem severity: gambling frequency $r = 0.39$; highest amount gambled in one day $r = 0.42$; current gambling debt $r = 0.47$; number of financial problems $r = 0.40$; number of borrowing sources $r = 0.31$; and legal problems $r = 0.50$	NA

Instrument	Content areas	Number of items	Administration time and method
Adult Instruments for Screening and Diagnosis *(continued)*			
National Opinion Research Center DSM-IV Screen for Gambling Problems (NODS) (National Opinion Research Center 1999)	DSM-IV diagnostic criteria for diagnosing PG, including lifetime and past-year time frames; a filtering question of losing $100 or more was used before administration of NODS	17	5- to 10-min interview
Lie/Bet Questionnaire (Johnson et al. 1997)	Lie to people about one's gambling; bet more and more money	2	1-min interview
Gambling Assessment Module (GAM-IV) (Cunningham-Williams et al. 2003)	Gambling frequency and DSM-IV diagnostic criteria for 11 different gambling activities	12 items administered separately for 11 different types of gambling behavior	Interview or self-administered

| Scoring | Psychometrics | | Classification accuracy indices |
	Reliability[†]	Validity	
1 point is scored for each DSM criterion Score range: 0–10 0=low-risk gambler 1 or 2=at-risk gambler 3 or 4=problem gambler 5+=pathological gambler	2- to 4-wk TRT coefficients of $r=0.99$ (lifetime) and $r=0.98$ (past year)	Administered to 40 individuals in outpatient problem gambling treatment programs Of 40 subjects, 38 scored 5+ on lifetime NODS; 2 obtained scores of 4 For past-year NODS, 30 scored 5+, 5 scored 3 or 4, and 5 scored 2 or less	NA
Answering yes to one or both items indicates PG	NA	NA	Computed on 191 male GA members and 171 male nonproblem gambling control subjects; Sens=0.99, Spec=0.91, PPV=0.92, and NPV=0.99 A second study that included females reported Sens=1.00, Spec=0.85, PPV=0.78, and NPV=1.00
A score of 5+ indicates PG	NA	Concordance with clinician ratings was fair for five diagnostic criteria ($\kappa=0.5-0.7$) and poor for other five criteria ($\kappa=0.0-0.3$).	NA

Instrument	Content areas	Number of items	Administration time and method
Adult Instruments for Screening and Diagnosis *(continued)*			
Gambling Behavior Interview (GBI) (Stinchfield et al. in press)	Clinical interview to measure signs and symptoms of PG, including gambling frequency, amount of time and money spent gambling, SOGS, DSM-IV, and 32 research items with a past-year time frame	76, including 20 SOGS, 10 DSM-IV diagnostic criteria, and 32 research items	30- to 60-min interview

	Psychometrics		
	---	---	
Scoring	**Reliability†**	**Validity**	**Classification accuracy indices**

Scoring	Reliability†	Validity	Classification accuracy indices
DSM score of 5+ indicates PG 20-item research scale uses item weights 5-item screen score of 2+ indicates probable PG	DSM-IV, α=0.95 20-item research scale, α=0.96 5-item screen, α=0.95	20-item research scale and 5-item screen correlated with DSM-IV diagnostic criteria scale (r=0.90; r=0.92), and with SOGS score (r=0.82; r=0.85)	Group membership was criterion: gambling treatment patients (n=121) and members of general population who had gambled in past year (n=138) Classification accuracy was computed for discriminating between the two groups; BR=0.47 DSM-IV using standard cutoff score of 5+: ODA=0.91; Sens=0.83; Spec=0.98; FPR=0.03; and FNR=0.13 20-item research scale using item weights yielded the following accuracy indices: ODA=1.00; Sens=1.00; Spec=1.00; FPR=0.00; and FNR=0.00 5-item screen with cutoff score of 2+: ODA=0.99; Sens=0.99; Spec=0.99; FPR=0.02; and FNR=0.01

Instrument	Content areas	Number of items	Administration time and method
Adult Instruments for Screening and Diagnosis *(continued)*			
Early Intervention Gambling Health Test (EIGHT) (Sullivan 1999)	Problem gambling signs and symptoms	8	5 min; questionnaire or interview
Time-Line Follow-Back (TLFB) and TLFB adapted for gambling (G-TLFB) (Stinchfield et al. 2001; Hodgins and Makarchuk 2003)	A calendar to measure gambling days and money spent gambling	Adapted for different time periods: 1 year, 6 months, or past 4 wks	Number of items varies by time period assessed
Addiction Severity Index–Pathological Gamblers (ASI-PG) and Gambling Severity Index (GSI) (Lesieur and Blume 1992)	Modification of ASI for pathological gamblers by adding items on gambling frequency and problems associated with gambling	6 items in GSI	Additional 10 min to administer gambling items
Structured Clinical Interview for Pathological Gambling (SCI-PG) (Grant et al., in press)	DSM-IV diagnostic criteria for PG	11 items cover 10 inclusion criteria and 1 exclusion criterion	15-min clinician-administered interview

| | **Psychometrics** | | |
Scoring	**Reliability†**	**Validity**	**Classification accuracy indices**
Each item=1 point Cutoff score of 4+ indicates that gambling is affecting patient's health	NA	Correlated with SOGS (r=0.75) Good to excellent with counselor ratings and diagnosis	Prison inmate sample (N=100) Compared with DSM-IV diagnosis: Sens=0.91; Spec=0.50 and PPV=0.59
Count days of gambling and days abstinent Sum the amount of time spent gambling; sum the amount of money lost gambling	3-wk TRT reliability: ICC=0.61–0.98; 2-wk TRT reliability: r=0.74–0.96	Agreement with collaterals: ICC=0.46–0.65 TLFB was correlated with other measures of gambling frequency (r=53) G-TLFB was correlated with SOGS (r=0.30); MAGS (r=0.28)	NA
Composite score range: 0–1 No specific interpretations given for scores; however, it is comparable to ASI indices	α=0.73	Correlation with SOGS (r=0.57)	NA
Diagnosis of PG is made if 5+ inclusionary questions and the exclusionary question are answered affirmatively	Interrater reliability: κ=1.00; 1-wk TRT reliability: κ=1.00 and r=0.97	Concurrent validity: correlation with SOGS (r=0.78) Discriminant validity: correlation with measure of anxiety (r=0.23) and depression (r=0.19)	SCI-PG diagnosis compared with longitudinal assessment: Sens=0.88; Spec=1.00; PPV=1.00; NPV=0.67

Instrument	Content areas	Number of items	Administration time and method
Adult Instruments for Evaluation and Treatment Efficacy			
Gambling Treatment Outcome Monitoring System (GAMTOMS) (Stinchfield and Winters 1996)	GTAQ includes 10-item measure of DSM-IV diagnostic criteria for PG and other measures of gambling problem severity, including SOGS, gambling frequency, gambling-related financial problems, and legal problems	142-item GTAQ with 10-item measure of DSM-IV diagnostic criteria	30- to 45-min PPQ
Pathological gambling modification of the Yale-Brown Obsessive-Compulsive Scale (PG-YBOCS) (Hollander et al. 1998)	Assesses change in gambling symptoms; includes 5-item Urges/Thought subscale and 5-item Behavior subscale	10	15- to 30-min clinician-administered interview
Gambling Symptom Assessment Scale (G-SAS) (Kim et al. 2001)	Assesses change in gambling symptoms, including urges to gamble and thoughts associated with gambling	12	15- to 30-min self-report

| | Psychometrics | | |
Scoring	Reliability[†]	Validity	Classification accuracy indices
DSM-IV diagnostic criteria items are 1 point each and are summed. Score range: 0–10 Score of 5+ indicates PG	Internal consistency reliability: DSM-IV diagnostic criteria (α=0.89), SOGS (α=0.85), and financial problems (α=0.78) 1-wk TRT yielded correlations of r=0.74 (DSM-IV) and r=0.91(SOGS)	Validity of DSM-IV diagnostic criteria was measured by correlations with the following measures of gambling problem severity: SOGS (r=0.83); gambling frequency (r=0.43); and number of financial problems (r=0.40)	DSM-IV diagnosis of PG was used to classify clinical vs. nonclinical cases: BR=0.20; ODA=0.96; Sens=0.96; Spec=0.95; FPR=0.01; and FNR=0.14 DSM-IV diagnosis of PG was used to classify SOGS probable PG vs. non–probable PG cases: BR=0.79; ODA=0.98; Sens=0.97; Spec=1.00; FPR=0.00; and FNR=0.10
Response options range from 0 to 4; responses are summed Total score range: 0–40	Interrater agreement on Urges, ICC=0.99; on Behavior, ICC=0.98	Correlated with Clinical Global Impressions (CGI) (r=0.89) and SOGS (r=0.86)	NA
Response options range from 0 to 4; responses are summed Total score range: 0–48 Scores >30 are interpreted as severe; 21–30 as moderate; and <21 as mild	Internal consistency reliability: α=0.89; 1-wk TRT reliability: r=0.70	Correlated with CGI Improvement score (r=0.78) and Severity score (r=0.81)	NA

Instrument	Content areas	Number of items	Administration time and method
Adult Instruments for Evaluation and Treatment Efficacy *(continued)*			
Pathological gambling modification of Clinical Global Impressions (PG-CGI) Scale (Guy 1976)	Adapted for gambling; measures severity of illness, improvement, and therapeutic effect of drug	3	Clinician rates patient on 3 items in <5 min; patient can also do self-rating
Youth Instruments for Assessment			
South Oaks Gambling Screen–Revised for Adolescents (SOGS-RA) (Winters et al. 1993, 1995)	Signs and symptoms of problem gambling, negative consequences	12	10-min PPQ
DSM-IV Multiple Response–Juvenile (DSM-IV-MR-J) (Fisher 2000a)	DSM-IV diagnostic criteria for PG	9	5- to 10-min PPQ

Note. BR=base rate; FNR=false-negative rate; FPR=false-positive rate; GTAQ=Gambling Treatment Admission Questionnaire; ICC=internal conversion coefficient; NA=not available or not applicable; NPV=negative predictive value; ODA=overall diagnostic accuracy; PG=pathological gambling; PPQ=paper-and-pencil questionnaire; PPV=positive predictive value; Sens=sensitivity; Spec=specificity; TRT=test-retest.
[†]All instances of α refer to Cronbach α.

| | Psychometrics | | |
Scoring	Reliability[†]	Validity	Classification accuracy indices
7-point response options— Severity: 1 = not at all ill to 7 = extremely ill Improvement: 1 = very much improved to 7 = very much worse	NA	NA	NA
Each item = 1 point Score range: 0–12 0–1 = no problem 2–3 indicates "at risk" gambling 4 or more indicates problem gambling	$\alpha = 0.80$	Gambling activity ($r=0.39$); gambling frequency ($r=0.54$)	NA
Each item = 1 point Score range: 0–9 Score of 4 or more indicates problem gambling	$\alpha = 0.75$	Significantly different mean scores between regular and nonregular gamblers and between problem and social gamblers DSM-IV-MR-J problem gamblers also tended to play more games regularly, spend more money, borrow to fund their gambling, and sell their possessions to fund their gambling	NA

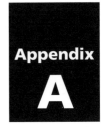

Appendix

A

DSM-IV-TR Criteria for Pathological Gambling

Source. Reprinted from American Psychiatric Association: *Diagnostic and Statistical Manual of Mental Disorders*, 4th Edition, Text Revision. Washington, DC, American Psychiatric Association, 2000. Used with permission.

DSM-IV-TR Criteria for Pathological Gambling

A. Persistent and recurrent maladaptive gambling behavior as indicated by five (or more) of the following:

    (1) is preoccupied with gambling (e.g., preoccupied with reliving past gambling experiences, handicapping or planning the next venture, or thinking of ways to get money with which to gamble)

    (2) needs to gamble with increasing amounts of money in order to achieve the desired excitement

    (3) has repeated unsuccessful efforts to control, cut back, or stop gambling

    (4) is restless or irritable when attempting to cut down or stop gambling

    (5) gambles as a way of escaping from problems or of relieving a dysphoric mood (e.g., feelings of helplessness, guilt, anxiety, depression)

    (6) after losing money gambling, often returns another day to get even ("chasing" one's losses)

    (7) lies to family members, therapist, or others to conceal the extent of involvement with gambling

    (8) has committed illegal acts such as forgery, fraud, theft, or embezzlement to finance gambling

    (9) has jeopardized or lost a significant relationship, job, or educational or career opportunity because of gambling

    (10) relies on others to provide money to relieve a desperate financial situation caused by gambling

B. The gambling behavior is not better accounted for by a Manic Episode.

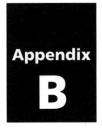

Early Intervention Gambling Health Test (EIGHT)

Source. Developed by Sean Sullivan, Ph.D., for the Compulsive Gambling Society of New Zealand Inc. and the Department of General Practice and Primary Health Care at the Auckland School of Medicine, 1999. Permission to republish granted by Dr. Sean Sullivan.

Early Intervention Gambling Health Test (EIGHT)

> Most people enjoy gambling, whether it's the lottery, sports, cards, bingo, racing, or at the casino.
> *Sometimes however it can affect our health.*
> To help us to check your health, please answer the questions below as truthfully as you are able from your own experience.

1. Sometimes I've felt depressed or anxious after a session of gambling.
   ____ Yes, that's true.　　　　____ No, I haven't.

2. Sometimes I've felt guilty about the way I gamble.
   ____ Yes, that's so.　　　　____ No, that isn't so.

3. When I think about it, gambling has sometimes caused me problems.
   ____ Yes, that's so.　　　　____ No, that isn't so.

4. Sometimes I've found it better not to tell others, especially my family, about the amount of time or money I spend gambling.
   ____ Yes, that's true.　　　　____ No, I haven't.

5. I often find that when I stop gambling I've run out of money.
   ____ Yes, that's so.　　　　____ No, that isn't so.

6. Often I get the urge to return to gambling to win back losses from a past session.
   ____ Yes, that's so.　　　　____ No, that isn't so.

7. Yes, I have received criticism about my gambling in the past.
   ____ Yes, that's true.　　　　____ No, I haven't.

8. Yes, I have tried to win money to pay debts.
   ____ Yes, that's true.　　　　____ No, I haven't.

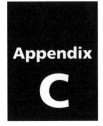

Gambling Symptom Assessment Scale (G-SAS)

Source. Reprinted from Kim SW, Grant JE, Adson DE, et al: "Double-Blind Naltrexone and Placebo Comparison Study in the Treatment of Pathological Gambling." *Biological Psychiatry* 49:914–921, 2001. Used with permission from Society for Biological Psychiatry and Elsevier.

Gambling Symptom Assessment Scale (G-SAS)

The following questions are aimed at evaluating gambling symptoms. Please *read* the questions *carefully* before you answer.

1. **If you had urges to gamble during the past WEEK, on average, how strong were your urges? Please circle the most appropriate number.**

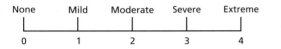

2. **During the past WEEK, how many times did you experience urges to gamble? Please circle one.**
   0) None
   1) Once
   2) Two to three times
   3) Several to many times
   4) Constant or near constant

3. **During the past WEEK, how many hours (add up hours) were you preoccupied with your urges to gamble? Please circle the most appropriate number.**

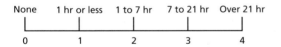

4. **During the past WEEK, how much were you able to control your urges? Please circle the most appropriate number.**

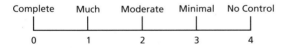

5. **During the past WEEK, how often did thoughts about gambling and placing bets come up? Please circle the most appropriate number.**

   0) None
   1) Once
   2) Two to three times
   3) Several to many times
   4) Constantly or nearly constantly

6. During the past WEEK, approximately how many hours (add up hours) did you spend thinking about gambling and thinking about placing bets? Please circle the most appropriate number.

```
None    1 hr or less   1 to 7 hr    7 to 21 hr   Over 21 hr
 |           |            |            |            |
 0           1            2            3            4
```

7. During the past WEEK, how much were you able to control your thoughts about gambling? Please circle the most appropriate number.

```
Complete      Much      Moderate     Minimal    No Control
 |             |           |            |            |
 0             1           2            3            4
```

8. During the past WEEK, approximately how much total time did you spend gambling or on gambling related activities? Please circle the most appropriate number.

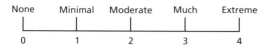

```
None    2 hr or less   2 to 7 hr    7 to 21 hr   Over 21 hr
 |           |            |            |            |
 0           1            2            3            4
```

9. During the past WEEK, on average, how much anticipatory tension and/or excitement did you have shortly before you engaged in gambling? If you did not actually gamble, please estimate how much tension and/or excitement you believe you would have experienced, if you had gambled. Please circle the most appropriate number.

```
None     Minimal    Moderate      Much       Extreme
 |          |           |            |            |
 0          1           2            3            4
```

10. During the past WEEK, on average, how much excitement and pleasure did you feel when you won on your bet? If you did not actually win at gambling, please estimate how much excitement and pleasure you would have experienced if you had won. Please circle the most appropriate number.

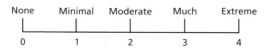

```
None     Minimal    Moderate      Much       Extreme
 |          |           |            |            |
 0          1           2            3            4
```

11. During the past WEEK how much emotional distress (mental pain or anguish, shame, guilt, embarrassment) has your gambling caused you? Please circle the most appropriate number.

None	Mild	Moderate	Severe	Extreme
0	1	2	3	4

12. During the past WEEK, how much personal trouble (relationship, financial, legal, job, medical or health) has your gambling caused you? Please circle the most appropriate number.

None	Mild	Moderate	Severe	Extreme
0	1	2	3	4

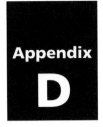

South Oaks
Gambling Screen (SOGS)

Source. Copyright 1992, South Oaks Foundation, reprinted by permission.
Lesieur HR, Blume SB: "The South Oaks Gambling Screen (SOGS): A New Instrument for the Identification of Pathological Gamblers." *American Journal of Psychiatry* 144:1184–1188, 1987; Lesieur HR, Blume SB: "Revising the South Oaks Gambling Screen in Different Settings." *Journal of Gambling Studies* 9:213–223, 1993

South Oaks Gambling Screen (SOGS)

1. Please indicate which of the following types of gambling you have done in your lifetime. For each type, mark only one answer: "not at all," "less than once a week," or "once a week or more."

	Not at all	Less than once a week	Once a week or more	
a.	____	____	____	Played cards for money
b.	____	____	____	Bet on horses, dogs or other animals (off-track betting, at the track, or with a bookie)
c.	____	____	____	Bet on sports (parlay cards, with a bookie, or at jai alai)
d.	____	____	____	Played dice games (craps, over and under, or other dice games) for money
e.	____	____	____	Went to casino (legal or otherwise)
f.	____	____	____	Played the numbers or bet on lotteries
g.	____	____	____	Played bingo
h.	____	____	____	Played the stock and/or commodities market
i.	____	____	____	Played slot machines, poker machines, or other gambling machines
j.	____	____	____	Bowled, shot pool, played golf, or played some other game of skill for money

2. What is the largest amount of money you have ever gambled with on any one day?

____ Never have gambled   ____ More than $10, up to $100

____ $1 or less   ____ More than $100, up to $1,000

____ More than $1, up to $10   ____ More than $1,000, up to $10,000

3. Do (did) your parents have a gambling problem?

____ Both my father and mother gamble (gambled) too much.

____ My father gambles (gambled) too much.

____ My mother gambles (gambled) too much.

____ Neither parent gambles (gambled) too much.

4. When you gamble, how often do you go back another day to win back money you lost?

____ Never

____ Some of the time (less than half the time) I lost

____ Most of the time I lost

____ Every time I lost

5. Have you ever claimed to be winning money gambling but weren't really?

____ Never (or never gamble)

____ Yes, less than half the time I lost

____ Yes, most of the time

6. Do you feel you have ever had a problem with gambling?

   ____ No

   ____ Yes, in the past, but not now

   ____ Yes

Check **Yes** or **No** for Questions 7–16   **Yes No**

7. Did you ever gamble more than you intended to?   ____ ____

8. Have people criticized your gambling?   ____ ____

9. Have you ever felt guilty about the way you gamble or what happens when you gamble?   ____ ____

10. Have you ever felt like you would like to stop gambling but didn't think you could?   ____ ____

11. Have you ever hidden betting slips, lottery tickets, gambling money, or other signs of your gambling from your spouse, children, or other important people in your life?   ____ ____

12. Have you ever argued with people you live with over how you handle money?   ____ ____

13. If you answered **Yes** to Question #12: Have money arguments ever centered on your gambling?   ____ ____

14. Have you ever borrowed from someone and not paid him or her back as a result of your gambling?   ____ ____

15. Have you ever lost time from work or school due to gambling?   ____ ____

16. If you borrowed money to gamble or to pay gambling debts, who or where did you borrow it from? Check **Yes** or **No** for each.

   a. from household money   ____ ____

   b. from your spouse   ____ ____

   c. from other relatives or in-laws   ____ ____

   d. from banks, loan companies or credit unions   ____ ____

   e. from credit cards   ____ ____

   f. from loan sharks (shylocks)   ____ ____

   g. You cashed in stocks, bonds or other securities.   ____ ____

   h. You sold personal or family property.   ____ ____

   i. You borrowed on your checking account (passed bad checks).   ____ ____

   j. You have (had) a credit line with a bookie.   ____ ____

   k. You have (had) a credit line with a casino.   ____ ____

SOGS Scoring

Scores on the South Oaks Gambling Screen itself are determined by adding up the number of questions that show an "at risk" response:

Questions 1, 2 and 3 are **not** counted.

___#4: Most of the time I lost **or** Every time I lost

___#5: Yes, less than half the time I lost **or** Yes, most of the time

___#6: Yes, in the past, but not now **or** Yes

___#7: Yes

___#8: Yes

___#9: Yes

___#10: Yes

___#11: Yes

Question 12 is **not** counted.

___#13: Yes

___#14: Yes

___#15: Yes

___#16a: Yes

___#16b: Yes

___#16c: Yes

___#16d: Yes

___#16e: Yes

___#16f: Yes

___#16g: Yes

___#16h: Yes

___#16i: Yes

Questions 16j and 16k are **not** counted.

Total = _____ (20 questions are counted.)

A total score of 5 or more = probable pathological gambler.

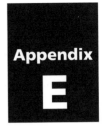

Yale-Brown Obsessive-Compulsive Scale Modified for Pathological Gambling (PG-YBOCS)

Source.   Reprinted with permission from Hollander E et al.

Reprinted from DeCaria CM, Hollander E, Begaz T, et al: "Reliability and Validity of a Pathological Gambling Modification of the Yale-Brown Obsessive Compulsive Scale (PG-YBOCS): Preliminary Findings." Presented at the 12th National Conference on Pathological Gambling. Las Vegas, NV, July 1998. Used with permission.

Yale-Brown Obsessive Compulsive Scale Modified for Pathological Gambling (PG-YBOCS)

1. Time occupied by urges/thoughts about gambling
How much of your time is occupied by urges/thoughts (u/t) related to gambling and/or gambling-related activities? How frequently does this occur?

0 = None
1 = Mild (less than 1 hr/day) or occasional u/t (≤8x/day)
2 = Moderate (1–3 hrs/day) or frequent u/t (≥8x/day but most hrs/day are free of u/t)
3 = Severe (>3 and up to 8 hrs/day) or very frequent u/t (>8x/day and occur most hrs of day)
4 = Extreme (>8 hrs/day) or near constant u/t (too numerous to count and an hour rarely passes w/o several such u/t occurring)

2. Interference due to urges/thoughts about gambling
How much do your urges/thoughts (u/t) interfere with your social or work (or role) functioning? Is there anything that you do not do because of this? (If patient is currently not working, determine how much performance would be affected if patient were employed.)

0 = None
1 = Mild, slight interference with social or occupational activity but overall performance is not impaired
2 = Moderate, definite interference with social or occupational performance, but manageable
3 = Severe, causes substantial impairment in social or occupational performance
4 = Extreme, incapacitating

3. Distress associated with urges/thoughts about gambling
How much distress do your urges/thoughts about gambling cause you? (Rate "disturbing" feeling or anxiety that seems to be triggered by these thoughts, not generalized anxiety or anxiety symptoms associated with other symptoms.)

0 = None
1 = Mild, infrequent and not too disturbing
2 = Moderate, frequent and disturbing, but still manageable
3 = Severe, very frequent and very disturbing
4 = Extreme, near constant and disabling distress

4. **Resistance against urges/thoughts of gambling**
How much of an effort do you make to resist these urges/thoughts?
How often do you try to disregard them? (Only rate effort made to resist, not success or failure in actually controlling these thoughts. How much one resists the urges/thoughts may or may not correlate with ability to control them.)

0 = Makes effort always to resist; symptoms so minimal doesn't need to actively resist
1 = Tries to resist most of the time
2 = Makes some effort to resist
3 = Yields to all such urges/thoughts without attempting to control them but does so with some reluctance
4 = Completely and willingly yields to all such urges/thoughts

5. **Degree or control over urges/thoughts about gambling**
How much control do you have over urges/thoughts about gambling?
How successful are you in stopping or diverting these urges/thoughts?

0 = Complete control
1 = Much control, usually able to stop/divert urges/thoughts with some effort and consideration
2 = Moderate control, sometimes able to stop/divert these urges/thoughts
3 = Little control, rarely successful in stopping these urges/thoughts, can only divert attention with difficulty
4 = No control, experienced as completely involuntary, rarely able to even momentarily divert urges/thoughts

6. **Time spent in activities related to gambling**
How much time do you spend in activities related to gambling? (directly related to gambling itself or activities such as negotiating financial transactions or searching for financial resources related to gambling)

0 = None
1 = Mild, spends less than 1 hr/day in these activities, or occasional involvement in these activities (≤8 times/day)
2 = Moderate (1–3 hrs/day) or >8 times/day but most hours are free of such activities
3 = Severe, spends >3 and up to 8 hrs/day or very frequent involvement (>8 times/day and activities performed most hours of the day
4 = Extreme (spends >8 hrs/day in these activities) or near constant involvement (too numerous to count and an hour rarely passes without engaging in several such activities)

7. Interference due to activities related to gambling

How much do the above activities interfere with your social/work (or role) functioning?

Is there anything that you do not do because of them? (If patient is currently not working, determine how much performance would be affected if patient were employed.)

0 = None

1 = Mild, slight interference with social or occupational activities, but overall performance is not impaired

2 = Moderate, definite interference with social/occupational performance, but still manageable

3 = Severe, causes substantial impairment in social/occupational performance

4 = Extreme, incapacitating

8. Distress associated with behavior related to gambling

How much distress do you feel if prevented from gambling? (Pause) How anxious would you become?

0 = None

1 = Mild, only slightly anxious if behavior is prevented or only slight anxiety during behavior

2 = Moderate, reports that anxiety would mount but remains manageable if behavior is prevented or that anxiety increases but remains manageable during such behaviors

3 = Severe, prominent and very disturbing increase in anxiety if behavior is interrupted or prominent and very disturbing increase in anxiety during the behavior

4 = Extreme, incapacitating anxiety from any intervention aimed at modifying activity or incapacitating anxiety develops during behavior related to gambling

9. Resistance against gambling

How much of an effort do you make to resist these activities? (How much the patient resists behaviors may or may not correlate with ability to control them.)

0 = Makes an effort to always resist, or symptoms so minimal does not need to actively resist

1 = Tries to resist most of the time

2 = Makes some effort to resist

3 = Yields to almost all of these behaviors without attempting to control them but does so with some reluctance

4 = Completely and willingly yields to all behaviors related to gambling

10. **Degree of control over gambling behavior**

How strong is the drive to gamble?

How much control do you have over the behaviors associated with gambling-related activities?

0 = Complete control

1 = Much control, experiences pressure to gamble, but usually able to exercise voluntary control over it

2 = Moderate control, strong pressure to gamble, must be carried to completion, can only delay with difficulty

3 = Little control, very strong drive to gamble, must be carried to completion, can only delay with difficulty

4 = No control, drive to gamble experienced as completely involuntary and overpowering, rarely able to even momentarily delay gambling activity

Gambling Urge/Thought Subtotal (Q1–Q5): _____

Gambling Behavior Subtotal (Q6–Q10): _____

Overall Total: _____

Index

Page numbers printed in **boldface** type refer to tables or figures.